Medicinal Mushrooms Secrets

Unlock the Power of Nature to Improve your Health

Johanna Westwood

© Copyright 2023 - All rights reserved.

No portion of this book may be reproduced in any form without written permission from the publisher or author, except as permitted by U.S. copyright law.

<u>Legal Notice:</u>
This book is copyright protected. This is only for personal use. You cannot amend, distribute, sell, use, quote or paraphrase any part or the content within this book without the consent of the author.

<u>Disclaimer Notice:</u>

This publication is designed to provide accurate and authoritative information in regard to the subject matter covered. It is sold with the understanding that neither the author nor the publisher is engaged in rendering legal, investment, accounting or other professional services. While the publisher and author have used their best efforts in preparing this book, they make no representations or warranties with respect to the accuracy or completeness of the contents of this book and specifically disclaim any implied warranties of merchantability or fitness for a particular purpose. No warranty may be created or extended by sales representatives or written sales materials. The advice and strategies contained herein may not be suitable for your situation. You should consult with a professional when appropriate. Neither the publisher nor the author shall be liable for any loss of profit or any other commercial damages, including but not limited to special, incidental, consequential, personal, or other damages.

Table of Contents

Introduction

Humans have a longstanding relationship with mushrooms, an association that stretches back to the earliest days of our species. Leveraged as a nutrient source, a fire-making tool, and an aspect of spiritual ceremonies, mushrooms have also secured a crucial spot in traditional healing systems globally. Nowadays, as contemporary science strives to unearth innovative therapies and optimize human health, investigators are uncovering the substantial medical potential these astonishing organisms hold.

Our quest commences by delving into the fundamental comprehension of what fungi represent—unpretentious yet intricate life forms that are neither flora nor fauna but stand as a kingdom in their own right. We delve into the annals of fungi's employment in medicine and nutrition, gleaning insights from assorted cultures and eras.

This work clarifies misconceptions surrounding fungi, offers a synopsis of their role in health and illness, and presents a categorization of medicinal mushrooms. It also examines the biological characteristics of therapeutic mushrooms and familiarizes readers with some prevalent varieties.

As we untangle the scientific discussion encircling medicinal mushrooms, you will discover detailed chapters on how mushrooms enhance immunity, their potential influence on neurological operations, and their anti-inflammatory and antioxidant traits. We examine the research on mushrooms' potential effects on lifespan, gut health, cardiac health, and even their possible role in cancer treatment.

You will encounter guidelines on how to process mushrooms for maximum benefits, understand the contrast between supplements and whole mushrooms, and learn about possible side effects and interactions. We also impart tips on incorporating mushrooms into an immune-boosting diet, an anti-aging regime, a gut-friendly diet, and a heart-healthy diet. Additionally, we'll acquaint you with some straightforward and nutritious mushroom recipes that you can experiment with at home.

This guide is designed to be an empowering instrument, endowing you with the knowledge required to make informed decisions about your health. As we clarify the science and excavate the wisdom of traditional practices, our aspiration is that you find motivation and practical counsel in these pages that guide you to a healthier, enriched existence.

Welcome to the path to better health!

Chapter One: The Basics

Fungi represent a remarkably varied and intriguing collection of life forms, each occupying their own distinct kingdom, setting them apart from the realms of both plants and animals. This kingdom encapsulates entities we encounter daily, such as mushrooms, yeast, and molds, and also includes those we rarely notice, like the sprawling networks of mycelium hidden beneath the earth's surface. Current research has recorded over 120,000 varieties of fungi, but speculative estimates suggest the existence of a whopping 5.1 million species in total.

The structural design of fungal cells sets them apart in the natural world. Unlike their botanical counterparts, cells of fungi are encased in a tough cell wall predominantly made up of chitin, a sophisticated polysaccharide also present in the hard external coverings of arthropods, including insects and crustaceans. This sharply contrasts with the cellulose-based cell walls of plants. Internally, fungal cells are equipped with a nucleus and other dedicated organelles, earmarking them as eukaryotes, a classification they share with animals and plants.

Fungi fall under the category of heterotrophs, implying they nourish themselves by absorbing nutrients from their surroundings rather than generating their own sustenance through photosynthesis, as plants do. They discharge enzymes which simplify complex organic materials into manageable components, which they subsequently absorb for their nourishment. This renders them indispensable recyclers in ecosystems, ensuring the decomposition of organic matter and facilitating the return of nutrients to the soil.

When it comes to reproduction, fungi employ an impressive range of methods. Many are capable of both sexual and asexual reproduction, dictated by the conditions of their environment. Spores, the primary means of fungal reproduction, possess remarkable resilience, enabling their survival in harsh conditions. They can be dispersed through the elements - wind and water, or transported by animals, granting fungi the capacity to inhabit new surroundings.

When we refer to the term "mushroom", we're generally speaking of the fruiting body of the fungus, responsible for producing and releasing spores. The major part of a fungus, however, consists of a delicate network of thread-like structures known as hyphae, which together form the mycelium. This mycelium usually resides out of sight in soil, wood, or other substrates, drawing nutrients and expanding until environmental conditions prompt the production of mushrooms.

While it's true that certain types of fungi can be detrimental (pathogenic), instigating diseases in plants, animals, and humans, there are many others that yield significant benefits. Among these are medicinal mushrooms, the subject of our present exploration. These have been harnessed for their wellness-boosting properties over centuries, particularly within the sphere of traditional Chinese medicine. These fungi are rich in bioactive compounds with a wide range of potential therapeutic benefits, from bolstering the immune system to demonstrating anti-cancer properties.

Brief History of Fungi in Medicine and Nutrition

The intriguing world of fungi, specifically the medicinal mushrooms, carries a rich and layered narrative, intertwined with the fields of healthcare and nutrition over millennia.

Documented instances of medicinal mushroom usage hark back to the traditional medical practices of China and Tibet. As far back as 450 BCE, particular mushrooms were mentioned in the Yellow Emperor's Classic of Internal Medicine, a cornerstone of Chinese medicinal texts. Of special mention was Ganoderma lucidum, better known as "Lingzhi" or "Reishi". This was deemed the mushroom of immortality, attributed to its alleged longevity-enhancing qualities.

In the sphere of traditional Chinese medicine, assorted species of medicinal mushrooms were used as remedies for diverse afflictions. For instance, Shiitake mushrooms (Lentinula edodes) were thought to promote digestion and invigorate Qi, the life energy coursing through the body.

Meanwhile, Cordyceps were lauded for their abilities to amplify stamina and combat weariness.

Parallelly, medicinal mushrooms found their place in Ayurveda, the age-old medical system prevalent in India. In this context, they were commonly employed to maintain equilibrium among the doshas, the trio of vital energies regulating physiological functions.

In contrast, the West did not readily acknowledge the healing potential of mushrooms until a much later period. It was only in the 20th century that Western medicine began to recognize the curative possibilities offered by fungi, leading to rigorous scientific explorations. The isolation of penicillin by Dr. Alexander Fleming in 1928, extracted from the mold Penicillium notatum, represented a momentous turning point in medical advancement. This ushered in the era of antibiotics, forever altering the course of medicine by introducing effective solutions for bacterial infections.

With regard to nutrition, mushrooms have been cherished for their culinary contributions for ages. They enjoyed high esteem among ancient Romans, who dubbed them "food of the gods", and Egyptians, who deemed them a treat worthy of monarchs. Beyond their distinctive taste and texture, mushrooms have been valued for their nutritive merits, encompassing substantial protein, essential vitamins and minerals, along with low fat and calorie content.

The previous several decades have seen a surge in the popularity of medicinal mushrooms. Contemporary scientific studies persist in unveiling a multitude of health-promoting effects associated with their intake, such as immune regulation, cancer prevention, and neuroprotection. This has sparked curiosity in these captivating organisms as a natural reservoir of therapeutic compounds.

Despite the long-standing tradition of medicinal mushroom use, we're only just beginning to fathom their extensive potential and the mechanisms underlying their health benefits. The narrative of these mushrooms is a blend of age-old wisdom and modern scientific corroboration, indicating that the keys to well-being might be concealed in the most unanticipated corners.

Misconceptions

As we explore the intriguing universe of medicinal mushrooms, it's crucial to rectify common inaccuracies about fungi, especially mushrooms. Such misconceptions frequently obstruct individuals from fully understanding and appreciating the profound benefits and diversity that the fungal world brings.

"Every mushroom is identical": This belief that all mushrooms are alike is significantly flawed. Mushrooms are part of the extensive and varied kingdom of life forms known as fungi. Within this realm, it's estimated that 2-4 million species of fungi exist, but merely around 10% have been officially classified. Each type of mushroom varies greatly in terms of size, color, shape, texture, habitat, and life cycle. Moreover, mushrooms have notable differences in their chemical makeup. Some mushrooms are suitable for eating and are a rich source of nutrients like vitamins, minerals, and proteins. Others have medicinal properties, housing bioactive elements that can deliver substantial health benefits. For instance, specific species of the Ganoderma genus are used in traditional medicine for their potential to fortify immune health. On the other hand, some mushrooms are toxic or psychoactive, comprising substances that can induce severe illness or altered mental states. Amanita phalloides, often referred to as the "death cap," is lethal if ingested, while Psilocybe cubensis is a species frequently associated with psychedelic experiences. Grasping the unique traits and properties of each mushroom species is essential, particularly for those keen on foraging or eating them.

"Mushrooms belong to the plant kingdom": This is a prevalent misunderstanding, but it's not accurate scientifically. Mushrooms are not plants; instead, they are members of a separate biological kingdom called Fungi. The separation between fungi and plants arises from their unique physiological and genetic attributes. Contrary to plants, which generate their own food via photosynthesis, mushrooms are heterotrophic, implying that they draw their nutrients from the environment, primarily from decomposing organic materials. Fungi, including mushrooms, have an essential role in ecosystems as decomposers and recyclers of organic matter. Also, at the cellular level, mushrooms contain chitin in their cell walls, a compound also present in the exoskeletons of insects and crustaceans, while plants have cellulose. Hence, despite mushrooms sometimes bearing a superficial resemblance to plants, they're fundamentally different in terms of their biology and ecological functions.

"Every mushroom is safe to eat": This notion is perilously incorrect. While a large number of mushrooms are indeed edible and savored globally for their unique taste and texture, a significant number are inedible or even fatal. The edibility of a mushroom is determined by its species. Some species, like Agaricus bisporus, which include familiar varieties such as button, cremini, and portobello mushrooms, are commonly consumed. Other species, like Morchella or the "morel" mushrooms, are coveted for their unique flavor. However, there exist many mushroom species that are poisonous and can trigger symptoms that range from gastrointestinal discomfort to organ failure and even death. Infamous examples comprise Amanita phalloides, known as the "death cap," and Amanita virosa, known as the "destroying angel." Both house deadly toxins that can cause severe poisoning if ingested. Consequently, one should never eat a mushroom unless it has been definitively identified as safe by a knowledgeable individual. For those intrigued by foraging for wild mushrooms, it's crucial to possess a thorough understanding of mushroom identification or to be escorted by a seasoned guide. Misidentification can result in grave, and sometimes fatal, repercussions.

"Mushrooms lack nutritional benefits": This belief is incorrect. Mushrooms can be a considerable source of nutrition, presenting a varied range of vitamins, minerals, and other essential nutrients, while maintaining low levels of calories and fat. They are an excellent source of protein, a crucial macronutrient needed for muscle development and repair, and dietary fiber, which aids in promoting digestive health. In addition, mushrooms provide a generous supply of essential vitamins and minerals. They house B vitamins, including riboflavin (B2), niacin (B3), and pantothenic acid (B5), which play key roles in energy production, DNA repair, and maintaining our nervous system's health. Furthermore, mushrooms are a significant source of the mineral selenium, beneficial for the immune system's health and acting as an antioxidant. Other minerals found in mushrooms include potassium, which assists in managing blood pressure, and copper, essential for producing red blood cells and preserving nerve cells. Uniquely, certain mushrooms, when exposed to sunlight or ultraviolet light, can offer vitamin D, a nutrient vital for bone health and immune function, and which isn't commonly found in many foods. Hence, incorporating mushrooms into a balanced diet can positively contribute to overall health and nutrition.

"Medicinal mushrooms are a recent trend": While it may appear that the use of medicinal mushrooms is a recent phenomenon, particularly with their rising presence in health and wellness markets, their usage can be traced back thousands of years. Societies around the globe, particularly in the realm of traditional Chinese medicine, have revered medicinal mushrooms for their health-enhancing properties. Species like Reishi (Ganoderma lucidum), Cordyceps (Cordyceps sinensis), and Lion's Mane (Hericium erinaceus) have been utilized in herbal medicine for ages to support various aspects of human health, from bolstering the immune system to improving cognitive function. Current science is now beginning to corroborate these traditional applications through rigorous investigations. Numerous studies have detected bioactive components in these mushrooms that can deliver anti-inflammatory, immunomodulatory, anticancer, and neuroprotective effects, among other advantages. Thus, far from being a transient fashion, medicinal mushrooms have a lengthy history of application, and their recognition in the health and wellness sphere continues to rise with the progress of scientific research.

"Mushrooms are only consumed for their hallucinogenic effects": While it is accurate that certain mushrooms, such as those in the Psilocybe genus, comprise psychoactive elements and are renowned for their mind-bending effects, mushroom usage extends far beyond this. Many mushroom species lack psychoactive properties and are instead exploited for their culinary or medicinal benefits. Edible mushrooms, like button mushrooms (Agaricus bisporus) or shiitake mushrooms (Lentinula edodes), are eaten worldwide for their unique flavor and texture, and as mentioned before, they offer considerable nutritional value. Medicinal mushrooms, as already stated, have an extensive history in traditional medicine, with contemporary research validating their potential advantages for immune health, brain health, and more. It's important to note that the mushroom world is incredibly varied, with thousands of species each presenting its unique properties and uses. The focus on mushroom consumption is not confined to psychoactive experiences but encompasses a broad spectrum of applications, from culinary enjoyment to health enhancement.

These misconceptions serve to highlight the importance of education and awareness about the fascinating world of fungi. As research continues to unfold, we are increasingly recognizing fungi's vast potential, breaking down misconceptions, and acknowledging their crucial role in our ecosystems and health.

The Scope of Fungi in Health and Disease

Fungi, notably medicinal mushrooms, have a crucial part to play in both boosting wellbeing and tackling illness. Their invaluable contributions touch upon various dimensions of human health, including nourishment, immune response, mental wellbeing, and disease prevention and control.

Nourishment: Medicinal mushrooms stand out as an extraordinary source of nourishment, and they're often labelled as nutritional dynamos owing to their abundant supply of essential nutrients. They're loaded with vitamins such as B vitamins and Vitamin D. B vitamins, comprising B2 (riboflavin), B3 (niacin), and B5 (pantothenic acid), partake in an array of bodily functions, from bolstering skin health to facilitating cellular activities like energy generation. Vitamin D, a nutrient not typically found in many food items, plays a key part in calcium absorption, hence contributing to bone health and the operation of the immune system. Medicinal mushrooms also deliver a significant protein content, necessary for the formation and repair of body tissues, and fiber, which aids in digestion and helps regulate a healthy weight. Moreover, they house important minerals like selenium, possessing antioxidant qualities, and potassium, necessary for sustaining heart and muscle activity. Some mushrooms also have unique bioactive components, such as polysaccharides named beta-glucans, which have exhibited a variety of health-boosting effects, including strengthening the immune system and potentially lowering the risk of specific diseases. All these nutrients come with relatively low-calorie content, making medicinal mushrooms an extremely advantageous supplement to a well-rounded diet.

Immune Response: The immune-boosting effects of medicinal mushrooms are among their most celebrated attributes. Many of these mushrooms house compounds like beta-glucans, demonstrating immunomodulatory effects. Beta-glucans are complex sugars capable of sparking the immune system by activating specific immune cells such as macrophages and natural killer cells. These cells perform a crucial function in our body's defense system, aiding in the fight against pathogens and disease. By stimulating these cells, medicinal mushrooms enhance the body's immune response, bolstering its ability to ward off diseases and infections. Hence, routine consumption of these mushrooms can be a valuable companion in sustaining overall health and robustness.

Mental Wellbeing: In recent times, the capability of medicinal mushrooms to support brain health and mental wellness has drawn substantial attention. For example, Lion's mane mushroom (Hericium erinaceus) possesses bioactive elements that can trigger the production of nerve growth factor (NGF). NGF is a protein that has a key role in preserving and regenerating neurons, the cells that convey information in our brain. By boosting NGF, Lion's mane could potentially decelerate or even reverse cell degeneration in the brain. This suggests potential advantages for neurodegenerative conditions like Alzheimer's and Parkinson's disease. Additionally, this mushroom has been linked with reducing symptoms of anxiety and depression in certain studies, further hinting at its potential role in promoting mental health.

Disease Prevention and Management: Medicinal mushrooms, thanks to their array of bioactive substances, have shown promise in staving off and managing a variety of diseases. Studies have pointed towards potential anti-cancer, anti-diabetic, anti-viral, and anti-inflammatory attributes of these mushrooms. For example, the Turkey Tail mushroom (Trametes versicolor) is known to contain a substance known as polysaccharide-K (PSK), which has exhibited potential as a supplement to conventional cancer treatments. PSK appears to stimulate the immune system and restrain the proliferation of cancer cells, thereby potentially elevating survival rates in patients battling cancer. Similar research is underway with a range of other medicinal mushrooms, and while the need for additional research persists, the preliminary findings appear to hold promise.

Gastrointestinal Health: The wellbeing of our gut microbiome – the conglomerate of microorganisms residing in our digestive tract – plays a critical role in our overall health, with its influence extending from digestion to immunity to mood. Some mushrooms are categorized as prebiotics, substances that act as nourishment for advantageous gut bacteria. By catering to these beneficial bacteria, mushrooms can aid in maintaining a balanced gut microbiome, leading to a healthier digestive system. A well-balanced gut microbiome has been associated with a host of health benefits, including enhanced digestion, strengthened immune function, superior weight regulation, and even improved mental health owing to the connection between the gut and brain. It's becoming increasingly evident through research that many chronic health conditions, ranging from autoimmune diseases to mental health disorders, may be associated with imbalances in the gut microbiome. By integrating medicinal mushrooms, particularly those with prebiotic qualities, into our diet, we can foster a healthier and more balanced microbiome. This, in turn, could benefit overall health and wellbeing in a plethora of ways.

Despite these potential health advantages, it's imperative to bear in mind that medicinal mushrooms are not a cure-all or a replacement for a balanced diet, regular physical activity, sufficient rest, and professional healthcare. They should be viewed as an element of a comprehensive approach to health and wellbeing.

Chapter Two: A Brief Overview of Medical Mushrooms

Medicinal mushrooms, mirroring the expansive diversity within the realm of fungi, exhibit an array of varied attributes. With approximately 14,000 recognized mushroom species, only a handful are comprehensively understood and employed for their medicinal qualities. Here's an introduction to a few commonly known medicinal mushrooms (with examples):

Polypores

Ganoderma lucidum (Reishi or Lingzhi): Frequently referred to as the 'mushroom of eternal life' in time-honored Chinese manuscripts, Reishi has found use in traditional medicine spanning more than 2000 years. It is lauded for its potential abilities to modulate immune response. Reishi is rich in polysaccharides, including beta-glucans, and triterpenes, which are believed to bolster immune function by promoting the activity of immune cells and controlling inflammatory reactions. Various studies have also reported its anti-cancer properties, with its bioactive components potentially restricting the growth and inducing programmed cell death (apoptosis) in some cancer cells. Moreover, Reishi has been used in managing stress levels and improving sleep quality. Its triterpenes may potentially lessen symptoms of anxiety and depression, and elevate sleep quality, thereby attributing adaptogenic traits to the mushroom.

Trametes versicolor (Turkey Tail): Named for its vibrant, fan-shaped growth that resembles a turkey's tail, Turkey Tail is widely recognized for its potent effects on boosting immunity. It is rich in polysaccharides, particularly PSK (polysaccharide-K) and PSP (polysaccharide peptide), which are known to stimulate the immune system, activate certain immune cells, and boost the body's resilience against infections and diseases. PSK also exhibits potential anti-cancer properties. In Japan, it is used as a supplement to traditional cancer treatments like chemotherapy, with some studies suggesting it may enhance survival rates and improve the quality of life for cancer patients.

Grifola frondosa (Maitake): Translated as the 'dancing mushroom' in Japanese, Maitake is valued in traditional medicine for its myriad health benefits. Research posits that Maitake can support immune function, owing to its abundant content of beta-glucans. Furthermore, studies have indicated that Maitake could exhibit potential anti-diabetic attributes, potentially enhancing insulin sensitivity and hence aiding in controlling blood glucose levels. Its anti-cancer effects have also been investigated, with some research suggesting that Maitake extracts could inhibit the proliferation of certain types of cancer cells.

Gilled Mushrooms

Lentinula edodes (Shiitake): A staple in cuisines across the globe, Shiitake mushrooms bring more to the table than their distinct savory taste. They boast an abundant supply of polysaccharides, sterols, and lipids, which bolster their immune-enhancing and anti-viral capabilities. Shiitake mushrooms can fortify the immune system, improving its combat readiness against pathogens. They also contain a compound known as lentinan, demonstrating anti-viral potency against several viruses. Moreover, Shiitake mushrooms could potentially lower cholesterol levels, possibly by impeding cholesterol absorption in the gut, making them a heart-healthy choice.

Pleurotus ostreatus (Oyster Mushroom): Named for their resemblance to oysters, these mushrooms are not only easy to grow but are also packed with various health benefits. They are loaded with beta-glucans and other compounds possessing antioxidant capabilities, helping to ward off oxidative stress in the body. They've been researched for their potential anti-inflammatory effects, possibly achieved by curbing the production of pro-inflammatory molecules. Additionally, studies suggest that oyster mushrooms may possess cholesterol-lowering traits, which could be linked to their lovastatin content, a naturally occurring statin.

Tooth Fungi

Hericium erinaceus (Lion's Mane): Distinguished by its cascading spines instead of traditional mushroom caps, Lion's Mane has attracted interest due to its neuroprotective traits. This mushroom hosts hericenones and erinacines, compounds capable of inducing the production of nerve growth factor (NGF), a protein instrumental for the growth, upkeep, and survival of nerve cells. This points to the possibility of Lion's Mane potentially decelerating or reversing cell degeneration in the brain, thereby providing potential benefits for neurodegenerative conditions like Alzheimer's and Parkinson's disease. Besides, research indicates that Lion's Mane might support cognitive function, potentially enhancing memory and focus. Certain studies also suggest it may aid in alleviating symptoms of anxiety and depression.

Ascomycetes

Cordyceps sinensis (Caterpillar fungus): Known for its peculiar life cycle, where the fungus emerges from an insect host's body, Cordyceps has been employed in traditional Tibetan and Chinese medicine to boost stamina and fight fatigue, owing to its potential influence on increasing energy production at a cellular level. The mushroom has also been associated with improving respiratory health, possibly by promoting oxygen utilization and enhancing lung function, proving beneficial for conditions like asthma and chronic obstructive pulmonary disease (COPD). Moreover, Cordyceps has been traditionally used to improve sexual function, with some research suggesting potential enhancements in libido and erectile function.

Jelly Fungi

Tremella fuciformis (Snow Fungus): Also known as Silver Ear fungus, Snow Fungus has been a part of Chinese cuisine and medicine for many centuries. It is famed for its skin-enhancing properties, attributable to its rich polysaccharide content that can boost skin hydration and elasticity, potentially lessening wrinkles and other signs of skin aging. Beyond this, Snow Fungus showcases potent antioxidant properties that can assist in protecting cells against oxidative stress. Certain research has also suggested neuroprotective properties, with some extracts from Snow Fungus displaying potential protective effects against neurotoxicity and cognitive impairment in preclinical trials.

Biological Characteristics and Properties

Unique biological traits and bioactive ingredients differentiate mushrooms and lay the groundwork for their health-boosting capacities:

Biological Characteristics

Mycelium and Fruiting Bodies: A significant part of a mushroom's life cycle is devoted to the growth of mycelium, a complex system of minuscule, filamentous cells. This network can spread across extensive spaces, typically concealed within its substrate (such as wood or soil). When conditions are favorable (ideal temperature, humidity, and nutrient availability), the mycelium gives rise to fruiting bodies, what we commonly identify as mushrooms. These fruiting bodies serve a reproductive role, disseminating millions of spores that can disperse and colonize new regions.

Chitin Cell Walls: The cell walls of fungi, inclusive of medicinal mushrooms, consist of chitin, a sophisticated carbohydrate also present in the exoskeletons of insects and crustaceans. Humans lack the enzyme necessary to break down chitin, which is one reason why certain medicinal mushrooms are traditionally processed through cooking or extraction techniques to increase the bioavailability of their beneficial compounds.

Decomposers and Symbionts: Numerous mushrooms perform pivotal roles in ecosystems as decomposers, dismantling organic material and recycling nutrients back into the soil. Some form symbiotic alliances with plants, aiding in nutrient absorption in return for sugars. These ecological roles allude to their exceptional biochemical abilities.

Bioactive Properties

Polysaccharides: Several medicinal mushrooms produce intricate polysaccharides, such as beta-glucans, proven to possess potent immune-modulating effects. These compounds can stimulate the immune system, enabling it to function more efficiently.

Terpenoids: Specific mushrooms generate a variety of terpenoids, organic compounds often exhibiting strong biological activity. For instance, the triterpenoids present in Reishi mushrooms have been researched for their potential anti-inflammatory, antioxidant, and anti-cancer properties.

Proteins and Peptides: Some medicinal mushrooms generate unique proteins and peptides with bioactive properties. For example, the protein lentinan derived from Shiitake mushrooms has showcased anti-cancer effects in certain studies.

Antioxidants: Medicinal mushrooms are a rich reservoir of antioxidants, which can safeguard the body from harm caused by free radicals. This encompasses phenolic compounds, ascorbic acid (vitamin C), tocopherols (vitamin E), and carotenoids.

Vitamins and Minerals: Mushrooms are a valuable source of B vitamins (comprising riboflavin, niacin, and pantothenic acid), which bolster the nervous system and aid the body in breaking down proteins, fats, and carbohydrates for energy. They also offer minerals like selenium, potassium, and copper.

Effects can fluctuate based on the species, growth conditions, harvesting period, and preparation methods, highlighting the significance of quality when selecting medicinal mushroom products.

Legal and Ethical Considerations of Using Medicinal Mushrooms

The application of medicinal mushrooms introduces a myriad of legal and ethical points for consideration. Despite their increasing recognition as potential auxiliaries in health and wellness, regulatory structures, sustainability issues, and educated usage should be thoughtfully examined.

Regulatory Structures

The legality of medicinal mushrooms varies worldwide. In some areas, specific kinds of medicinal mushrooms are categorized as dietary supplements, while others are subject to more stringent regulations due to the presence of psychoactive compounds.

For instance, in the United States, most medicinal mushrooms are legally accessible as dietary supplements. However, certain substances like psilocybin, present in some mushroom species, are classified as Schedule I substances under the Controlled Substances Act, rendering them illegal to produce, distribute, or possess. Yet, this is evolving in some states where therapeutic use in controlled environments is permitted.

Hence, it's crucial to familiarize oneself with the laws in your country or state when contemplating the use of medicinal mushrooms, particularly those containing psychoactive substances.

Quality and Safety

With the escalating popularity of medicinal mushrooms, the market is inundated with products of varied quality. It's imperative to buy from trustworthy sources that guarantee their products are safe, effective, and devoid of contaminants like heavy metals or harmful microbes. This is where regulatory agencies play a role. For instance, in the U.S., the Food and Drug Administration (FDA) supervises dietary supplements, though it's worth mentioning that their regulation is less stringent than for pharmaceuticals.

Sustainability

The rising demand for medicinal mushrooms increases the strain on their natural environments. Excessive harvesting can lead to the exhaustion of wild mushroom populations and disrupt the ecosystems where they serve a crucial function. Hence, sustainable cultivation techniques and responsible foraging are essential to safeguard these precious resources for future generations.

Informed Use

While medicinal mushrooms can provide health advantages, they should not replace professional medical consultation or treatment. Individuals should seek advice from a healthcare provider before initiating any new supplement routine, especially those with pre-existing health issues or those who are pregnant or breastfeeding. Misuse can result in negative effects, or it might conflict with other treatments or medications. It's also essential to bear in mind that while research on medicinal mushrooms is encouraging, it's still in its infancy, and more comprehensive clinical trials are needed to fully comprehend their effects.

Chapter Three: The Immune-Enhancing Effects of Mushrooms

The immune system is a complex matrix of cells, tissues, and organs that collectively work to protect the body against harmful intruders such as bacteria, viruses, and cancerous cells. Recognizing the role of the immune system in health and disease is key to understanding the potential benefits of medicinal mushrooms, celebrated for their immune-boosting properties.

The immune system consists of two primary elements: the innate immune system and the adaptive immune system.

Innate Immune System: Also known as the nonspecific immune system, the innate immune system forms the first line of defense against foreign intruders. This system is "innate" as it is essentially in place from birth, offering general defense mechanisms that don't target specific invaders.

Physical barriers like the skin and the mucous membranes lining the respiratory, gastrointestinal, and urogenital tracts serve as the frontline defense. Designed to keep pathogens at bay, these barriers also employ active mechanisms such as producing antimicrobial substances and moving mucus via cilia to trap and expel invaders.

If a pathogen manages to penetrate these physical barriers, it confronts specialized immune cells like macrophages, neutrophils, and dendritic cells. These cells employ pattern recognition receptors to spot pathogen-associated molecular patterns (PAMPs) - shared structures present in various pathogens but absent in human cells. Recognizing a PAMP enables these cells to initiate a quick response, like swallowing the pathogen (a process termed phagocytosis), releasing enzymes to eradicate it, or creating signaling proteins (cytokines) that provoke inflammation to draw more immune cells to the infection site.

The innate immune system also deploys other defensive strategies like the complement system, a sequence of proteins in the blood that can earmark pathogens for elimination or assemble a membrane attack complex to directly kill certain bacteria and viruses. Although the innate immune system provides an essential rapid response to infection, it lacks the ability to precisely recognize and remember individual pathogens, which is a unique feature of the adaptive immune system.

Adaptive Immune System: Also referred to as the acquired or specific immune system, the adaptive immune system is a more specialized and sophisticated aspect of our immune response. While it takes longer to respond than the innate immune system, its power lies in its ability to target distinct pathogens and form a memory of the infection for more efficient responses in future encounters.

The adaptive immune system depends on lymphocytes - T cells and B cells - each having a unique role in the immune response. T cells, which mature in the thymus, are mainly accountable for cell-mediated immunity. Some T cells, termed cytotoxic T cells, can directly destroy infected cells.

Others, called helper T cells, assist in activating B cells and cytotoxic T cells.

B cells, which mature in the bone marrow, handle humoral immunity. Once activated, they can transform into plasma cells that generate antibodies. These antibodies are proteins that can identify and bind to specific antigens on the surface of pathogens. This binding can neutralize the pathogen, tag it for destruction by other immune cells, or activate the complement system.

The adaptive immune system's distinguishing feature is immunological memory. Once B and T cells encounter a specific antigen, some of them transform into memory cells. These long-lasting cells can quickly trigger a powerful immune response upon reencountering the same antigen, a concept that forms the basis of the effectiveness of vaccinations. By exposing the immune system to a harmless version of the pathogen or its antigens, vaccines stimulate the production of memory cells, readying the immune system for a swift and potent response if it ever encounters the actual pathogen.

Under normal circumstances, these two arms of the immune system work in concert to keep us healthy, responding to and neutralizing threats as they arise.

The Immune System in Disease

When the immune system becomes compromised or malfunctions, it can trigger a disease. This can transpire in multiple ways:

Immunodeficiency: A scenario where the immune system is less powerful than normal leaves the body susceptible to infections. This could be the consequence of genetic conditions like primary immunodeficiency diseases or external influences such as HIV/AIDS or certain kinds of cancer treatment.

Autoimmunity: Sometimes, the immune system erroneously combats the body's own cells, resulting in autoimmune diseases such as rheumatoid arthritis, type 1 diabetes, and lupus.

Chronic Inflammation: A robust immune response incorporates inflammation to aid in fighting off intruders and mending injured tissues. However, when inflammation turns chronic, it can contribute to diseases like heart disease, diabetes, cancer, and neurodegenerative disorders such as Alzheimer's disease.

Cancer: The immune system has a crucial role in detecting and eradicating abnormal cells that can transform into cancer. Nevertheless, some cancer cells can dodge the immune system and proliferate.

Medicinal mushrooms can influence the immune system in a variety of ways. They contain compounds like beta-glucans that can stimulate the activity of macrophages and natural killer cells, intensifying the body's innate immune response. Certain mushrooms also possess anti-inflammatory properties that can aid in controlling an overactive immune response, potentially beneficial in situations of chronic inflammation or autoimmunity.

In the context of cancer, certain mushrooms have been researched for their potential to boost the effectiveness of the immune system in recognizing and combating cancer cells. Some are also being investigated for their potential to alleviate the side effects of traditional cancer treatments, which often impair the immune system.

How Mushrooms Boost Immunity: The Biochemical Mechanisms

Medicinal mushrooms have been a staple in global traditional medicine practices for hundreds of years, and an expanding volume of scientific studies uphold their role in bolstering immune health. These fungi possess a unique assortment of compounds that can engage with our immune systems in numerous and intricate ways. Let's delve into some of the principal biochemical mechanisms through which mushrooms may enhance immunity:

Beta-Glucans

Beta-glucans are intricate polysaccharides found in the cell walls of bacteria, fungi, yeasts, and specific plants. Many medicinal mushrooms, such as Reishi, Shiitake, and Turkey Tail, are abundant sources of beta-glucans.

Within the body, beta-glucans are identified by various immune cells, including macrophages, neutrophils, and natural killer (NK) cells, through specific receptors like Dectin-1 and complement receptor 3 (CR3). Upon binding to these receptors, beta-glucans can stimulate a cascade of immune responses, including:

- Amplifying the phagocytic activity of macrophages, which improves their ability to consume and annihilate pathogens.

- Encouraging the production of cytokines, signaling molecules that regulate immune and inflammatory responses.

- Boosting the cytotoxic activity of NK cells, augmenting their ability to eliminate infected cells or cancer cells.

Terpenoids and Phenolic Compounds

Certain mushrooms produce terpenoids, organic compounds with a range of structures and functions. Some terpenoids, like triterpenoids discovered in Reishi mushrooms, have shown anti-inflammatory and antioxidant effects, potentially supporting immune health by curbing chronic inflammation and shielding cells from harm.

Similarly, mushrooms are loaded with phenolic compounds, which also have antioxidant properties. By neutralizing free radicals, these compounds can inhibit cellular damage and foster a healthy immune response.

Proteins and Peptides

Medicinal mushrooms can create a variety of proteins and peptides with immune-modulating properties. For instance, the protein lentinan from Shiitake mushrooms has demonstrated a stimulation of the immune response and is even recognized in Japan as an adjuvant for cancer therapy.

Myco-Nutrients

Mushrooms offer various vitamins and minerals that are crucial for immune function. For instance, they can provide copper, which participates in the development and function of immune cells; selenium, which assists in regulating inflammation; and vitamin D, which modulates innate and adaptive immune responses.

Research and Evidence on Mushrooms and Immunity

The connection between medicinal mushrooms and the immune system is an active domain of scientific exploration. Numerous investigations propose that specific mushroom species can adjust the immune system, though more stringent clinical trials are needed to comprehensively understand their impacts. Here's a glimpse at some of the evidence related to mushrooms and immunity:

Shiitake (Lentinula edodes): Shiitake mushrooms incorporate a compound known as lentinan, which is a form of beta-glucan. Studies indicate that lentinan can invigorate the immune system and potentially decelerate the expansion of certain cancer cells. A research paper published in the "Journal of the American College of Nutrition" discovered that regular intake of shiitake mushrooms boosted the performance of gamma delta T cells and natural killer T cells, which are integral components of the immune response.

Reishi (Ganoderma lucidum): Reishi is another mushroom renowned for its immune-adjusting properties. Its bioactive compounds encompass triterpenoids, polysaccharides, and peptidoglycans. Investigations suggest that these compounds can assist in regulating both the innate and adaptive immune systems, potentially impacting aspects like cytokine production and the operation of various immune cells. Additionally, Reishi has demonstrated anti-inflammatory properties, which might assist in handling conditions connected with chronic inflammation.

Maitake (Grifola frondosa): The beta-glucans in Maitake mushrooms are believed to energize the immune system and may possess anti-cancer attributes. A research study published in the "Annals of Translational Medicine" discovered that Maitake extract could stimulate the immune response in patients with breast cancer.

Turkey Tail (Trametes versicolor): Turkey Tail comprises a compound named polysaccharide-K (PSK), which has been authorized in Japan as an adjuvant for cancer therapy. Research indicates that PSK can activate the immune system and obstruct the expansion of specific cancer cells. A study published in "Global Advances in Health and Medicine" found that Turkey Tail could enhance immune functionality in patients suffering from breast cancer.

Cordyceps (Cordyceps sinensis): Traditionally utilized to elevate vitality and stamina, Cordyceps has also exhibited immune-adjusting properties. Studies suggest that it can encourage the production of specific immune cells and cytokines and potentially has anti-inflammatory impacts.

Integrating Mushrooms into an Immune-Boosting Diet

Infusing healing mushrooms into your everyday dishes not only introduces distinctive tastes but also helps you to reap numerous health benefits. Shiitake and Maitake are two examples of healing mushrooms that are prevalent in culinary use. Shiitake mushrooms, notable for their abundant and smoky taste, can be utilized in stir-fried dishes, soups, or as a replacement for meat. Maitake, with its tasty and faintly sweet tang, can be used similarly or even barbecued on its own. Preparing these mushrooms aids in breaking down their cell structure, improving the bioavailability of the nutrients and active compounds they enclose. When employing healing mushrooms in cuisine, it's critical to bear in mind that some mushrooms can incite adverse reactions when eaten raw, so it's advisable to ascertain they are properly prepared.

Mushroom Powders and Concentrates

For those who wish to amalgamate the advantages of healing mushrooms into their diet without cooking, mushroom powders and concentrates can be a fantastic alternative. They can effortlessly be incorporated into a variety of meals and beverages, including smoothies, coffee, soups, and even baked goods. For instance, Reishi mushroom, famous for its possible immune-stimulating and stress-reducing properties, is often ingested as a powder or concentrate due to its bitter taste when prepared. Similarly, Turkey Tail is generally consumed in concentrate form due to its tough texture. It's vital to ensure you select premium products from trusted brands that thoroughly test their products for strength and purity to circumvent potential pollutants or subpar quality products.

Mushroom Supplements

If you're pursuing a direct and handy way to infuse healing mushrooms into your health regimen, supplements can be a great choice. These are accessible in various forms, such as capsules, tablets, or liquid tinctures, each offering a concentrated dosage of the beneficial compounds found in healing mushrooms. Whether you're looking to fortify your immune system, boost cognitive function, or support overall wellbeing, there's likely a mushroom supplement that can assist. As always, it's crucial to adhere to the suggested dosages given by the manufacturer and consult a healthcare professional before initiating any new supplement regimen to ensure it's suitable for your individual health requirements and conditions.

Hybrid Approach

Employing a hybrid approach can be a beneficial strategy to acquire a wider spectrum of health benefits, as each variety of healing mushroom contains a unique profile of active compounds. For instance, you might take a Lion's Mane supplement for cognitive support, cook with Shiitake for cardiovascular health, and drink a Reishi tea for immune support. Additionally, numerous supplements in the marketplace merge several types of healing mushrooms, aiming to provide a comprehensive health boost by leveraging the combined effects of different mushrooms. This strategy, known as synergy, might amplify the benefits of individual mushrooms, offering a balanced and potent mix of health-supporting compounds.

Chapter Four: Mushrooms and Mental Health

The brain stands as the most intricate organ within the human form, acting as the central hub for the nervous system and facilitating cognition, memory, emotions, and perception. Additionally, it governs numerous biological operations, from the rhythm of the heart and respiration to hormone regulation. Mental health, on the other hand, covers our emotional, psychological, and social welfare and influences how we contemplate, experience emotions, behave, manage stress, engage with others, and make choices. Gaining insight into the brain and mental health is key when exploring the prospective advantages of healing mushrooms in these domains.

Basic Brain Structure and Function

The brain is segmented into multiple areas, each carrying out specialized tasks:

- The Brainstem manages fundamental survival operations like heart rhythm, respiration, and slumber.

- The Cerebellum coordinates deliberate movements, equilibrium, and muscle harmony.

- The Limbic System, which incorporates the hippocampus, amygdala, and hypothalamus, is accountable for emotions, long-term memory, and primary drives like hunger and carnal desire.

- The Cerebrum is partitioned into two halves and multiple lobes that oversee senses, motor function, reasoning, problem-solving, and other advanced cognitive abilities.

These regions are made up of billions of neurons that communicate using electrical signals and chemicals referred to as neurotransmitters, establishing complex networks that facilitate intricate brain functions.

Mental Health and Disorders

Mental health, often recognized as a state of overall wellness where a person can acknowledge their own capabilities, handle regular life stressors, carry out productive and rewarding work, and make a valuable contribution to their community. It's not only the lack of mental diseases but also encompasses emotional, psychological, and social welfare.

A variety of elements can impact mental health, including biological aspects such as genetics and the chemistry of the brain. Life experiences, including trauma or abuse, as well as wider social, cultural, and environmental factors, can also influence mental health. Mental health disorders, alternatively known as mental illnesses, are conditions that impact a person's thought process, emotions, behavior, or mood. They span from common disorders like depression and anxiety to more serious conditions like schizophrenia and bipolar disorder.

Depression is often identified by extended periods of sadness and lack of interest, while anxiety disorders appear as excessive worry or fear. Bipolar disorder is marked by extreme mood swings, alternating between manic highs and depressive lows. Schizophrenia is a serious disorder that impacts a person's ability to think, feel, and behave clearly. Post-traumatic stress disorder (PTSD) can develop after a person has undergone a traumatic event and can result in flashbacks, nightmares, and severe anxiety.

These mental health disorders often come with changes in brain function, including imbalances in neurotransmitters, leading to various symptoms affecting a person's daily life functionality.

The Role of Neurotransmitters

Neurotransmitters act as the body's chemical communicators. They send signals across the synaptic gap between neurons, which are specialized cells that process and transmit information in the brain. Imbalances in neurotransmitters can notably impact mood, sleep, focus, and overall mental health.

Serotonin, dopamine, and glutamate are three vital neurotransmitters associated with mental health. Serotonin, often called the 'feel-good' neurotransmitter, aids in the regulation of mood, sleep, appetite, and other important functions. Low serotonin levels are frequently associated with conditions like depression and anxiety.

Dopamine is another essential neurotransmitter that influences the brain's reward and pleasure centers and aids in the regulation of emotional responses. It's also responsible for motor coordination. Dysregulation of dopamine can lead to conditions like schizophrenia, marked by hallucinations and delusions, and addiction, characterized by an abnormal pursuit of reward.

Glutamate is the most abundant neurotransmitter and is involved in cognitive functions like learning and memory. An imbalance in glutamate is considered to contribute to a range of disorders, including OCD, autism, and major depression.

The Gut-Brain Axis and Mental Health

The term gut-brain axis refers to the physical and biochemical links between the gut and the brain. Recent discoveries have shown that the trillions of bacteria residing in our gut, collectively known as the gut microbiota, can impact brain function and behavior via this axis. This communication occurs through various pathways, including the vagus nerve, the immune system, stress hormones, and microbial metabolites.

Changes in the gut microbiota have been connected to various neurological and psychiatric disorders, including depression, anxiety, autism, and Parkinson's disease. This indicates that strategies to maintain a healthy gut microbiota may also support mental health. Such strategies might include a balanced diet rich in fiber and fermented foods, regular physical activity, adequate sleep, and probiotics, which are beneficial bacteria that can help balance the gut microbiota. However, more research is needed in this field to fully understand these connections and to develop effective interventions.

The Impact of Mushrooms on Neurological Processes

The potential influence of medicinal mushrooms on brain activities is a captivating area of scientific exploration. A myriad of studies propose that specific mushrooms contain biologically active compounds capable of interacting with our nervous system, potentially favoring brain health and emotional wellness. Here are some insights into how mushrooms might affect brain processes:

Neuroprotection

Neuroprotection refers to the measures and mechanisms adopted to shield the central nervous system (including the brain and spinal cord) from harm or damage that may arise from several causes. This concept is especially pertinent to conditions like Alzheimer's and Parkinson's, which involve the gradual impairment of neurons.

Various medicinal mushrooms harbor compounds demonstrated to showcase neuroprotective attributes. For instance, Lion's Mane (Hericium erinaceus), a mushroom recognized for its distinctive cascading spines, contains hericenones and erinacines. These compounds can trigger the creation of nerve growth factor (NGF), a protein essential for neuron health. By enhancing NGF levels, these compounds could potentially safeguard neurons from harm, potentially decelerating or reversing the progression of neurodegenerative disorders.

Reishi (Ganoderma lucidum), another mushroom with a long-standing history in traditional medicine, has also displayed potential for neuroprotection. Research suggests that compounds in Reishi can exert protective effects against neuronal damage, possibly via anti-inflammatory and antioxidant mechanisms. Similarly, Cordyceps (Cordyceps sinensis), an unusual mushroom that grows on insects, has shown neuroprotective capabilities, potentially enriching overall brain health.

Neurogenesis

Neurogenesis, the process of creating new neurons (nerve cells), is crucial for preserving cognitive function and mental health. Neurogenesis can be influenced by various factors, including diet, stress, physical activity, and sleep. It plays an essential role in learning, memory, and mood regulation.

Intriguingly, some medicinal mushrooms seem to support neurogenesis. For instance, Lion's Mane not only protects existing neurons - it might also stimulate the formation of new ones. This capability is tied to its influence on NGF levels. By boosting this crucial protein, Lion's Mane could potentially enhance cognitive function, improve mood, and lessen the effects of neurodegenerative disorders.

Modulation of Neurotransmitters

Chemical conveyors known as neurotransmitters relay signals within the brain, driving key brain functions such as emotional balance, cognitive ability, and response to stress. Disturbances in neurotransmitter levels can underpin mental health conditions.

Certain therapeutic fungi may hold the power to adjust neurotransmitter concentrations, potentially exerting influence over mental health. For instance, the mushroom Reishi has been the subject of research for its potential impacts on serotonin and dopamine, two pivotal neurotransmitters engaged in mood and reward regulation. Through affecting these neurotransmitters, Reishi may be capable of mood modulation, stress management, and bolstering mental wellness on the whole.

Support for the Gut-Brain Axis

The gut-brain pathway encompasses the bidirectional communication occurring between the gastrointestinal tract and the brain. It's become increasingly evident that a well-balanced gut microbial community, or gut microbiota, can have positive implications for brain health and operation.

Specific mushrooms such as Turkey Tail and Shiitake are recognized for bolstering a balanced gut microbiota. These mushrooms abound in prebiotic fibers like beta-glucans, which nourish the beneficial gut bacteria. By fostering a balanced gut microbiota, these mushrooms could influence the gut-brain pathway, potentially enhancing brain operation and mental health. For instance, a balanced gut microbiota has been associated with lower risks of mood disorders, enhanced cognitive function, and a more robust response to stress.

Mushrooms and Mood: Current Research

Hericium Erinaceus (Lion's Mane): The Lion's Mane mushroom is gaining research attention for its possible neuroenhancement abilities, especially its potential to boost nerve growth factor (NGF) production. NGF is a vital protein that fosters the growth, sustenance, and survival of neurons, thus playing an integral role in preserving the neural network. This attribute of Lion's Mane could conceivably be valuable in decelerating or reversing the progression of neurodegenerative disorders such as Alzheimer's and Parkinson's diseases.

Beyond its neuroprotective qualities, Lion's Mane might also hold benefits for mood balance. A small-scale study published in "Biomedical Research" in 2010 suggested that Lion's Mane intake lessened feelings of irritability and anxiety in women going through menopause. However, this study was not extensive and did not include a control group, thus requiring more wide-ranging research to definitively confirm these potential mood-enhancing effects.

Ganoderma Lucidum (Reishi): Contemporary research hints that Reishi could adjust levels of specific neurotransmitters, such as serotonin and dopamine, which are essential for mood balance, stress response, and overall mental wellness.

Initial animal studies have suggested potential anti-anxiety and antidepressant properties of Reishi. Yet, there is a shortage of comprehensive, large-scale human clinical trials that could definitively affirm these effects. Hence, while initial findings are hopeful, further research is needed to solidify the mood-enhancing benefits of Reishi in humans.

Cordyceps Sinensis and Cordyceps Militaris (Cordyceps): Cordyceps is recognized for its fatigue-reducing and energy-increasing properties. It has been traditionally employed to boost stamina and minimize stress. A study review published in the "Journal of Ethnopharmacology" in 2016 suggested that Cordyceps might have antidepressant-like properties in animals.

While these animal study findings are inspiring, human studies exploring the mood impacts of Cordyceps are relatively limited. Consequently, more research is needed to confirm its potential mood-enhancing effects in humans and to comprehend the mechanisms behind these effects.

Psilocybe Species (Psilocybin Mushrooms): Psilocybin, a psychoactive compound present in certain mushroom species, has been the subject of numerous clinical trials recently for its potential to treat various mental health disorders. Recent investigations have shown that, when used in a controlled and therapeutic setting, psilocybin can have substantial mood-boosting and antidepressant effects.

A noteworthy study published in "JAMA Psychiatry" in 2020 indicated that therapy assisted by psilocybin significantly ameliorated depressive symptoms in adults with major depressive disorder. However, it's crucial to acknowledge that psilocybin is a powerful psychoactive compound that should only be administered under the careful supervision of a medical professional, within the parameters of approved research or therapeutic protocols. Its use beyond these contexts can result in legal complications and health hazards.

Chapter Five: Mushrooms and Aging

Decoding the process of aging involves navigating through a web of various biological mechanisms. The two crucial elements that seem intricately connected to aging are inflammation and oxidative stress.

Oxidative stress arises when the equilibrium between the creation of free radicals (volatile molecules that can inflict harm to cells) and the body's competence to neutralize or cleanse their damaging effects is disrupted. This disproportion can culminate in cellular and tissue impairment, playing a part in the aging process and the onset of numerous age-associated ailments.

Free radicals can originate from typical metabolic processes or through external stimuli like pollutants, radiation, and toxins in our food and drink. The body is equipped with antioxidants, naturally present and obtained via diet, capable of neutralizing free radicals and shielding against their destructive effects.

As we age, the generation of free radicals can escalate while our antioxidant defenses might diminish, leading to heightened oxidative stress. This can inflict damage to cellular components such as DNA, proteins, and lipids, contributing to cellular senescence (the state of irreversible cell cycle cessation) and the onset of age-related illnesses such as cardiovascular disease, Alzheimer's disease, and cancer.

Inflammation plays a crucial role in the body's immune response to injury or infection. However, when inflammation becomes prolonged, it can contribute to an array of diseases and conditions, including aging.

The term "inflammaging" has been introduced to describe the low-grade persistent inflammation characteristic of aging. This inflammation can spur the generation of free radicals, thereby contributing to oxidative stress. It can also directly harm tissues and disrupt their standard functioning.

Numerous factors can contribute to inflammaging, including genetic predisposition, diet, lifestyle, exposure to toxins, and the accumulation of senescent cells, which secrete inflammatory substances.

Inflammaging has been implicated in many age-related diseases, such as cardiovascular disease, diabetes, cancer, Alzheimer's disease, and osteoarthritis.

Oxidative stress and inflammation establish an intricate, interdependent relationship within our bodies, each capable of provoking and exacerbating the other. In its essence, oxidative stress is a disequilibrium between the creation of free radicals (destructive, volatile molecules) and the body's capacity to neutralize or cleanse their damaging effects utilizing antioxidants. When this balance is skewed and free radicals become excessive, they can wreak havoc on cells, proteins, and DNA.

Our bodies mount an inflammatory response to shield against injuries and infections, but chronic inflammation can inflict significant damage. Oxidative stress can initiate inflammatory pathways, as cells under oxidative duress release signals to stimulate inflammation.

In contrast, the inflammatory response itself can create more free radicals, contributing to oxidative stress. This forms a destructive cycle that, if left unattended, can fuel the emergence and progression of various chronic diseases, such as heart disease, diabetes, neurodegenerative diseases like Alzheimer's, and cancer. The prolonged presence of oxidative stress and inflammation also correlates with accelerated aging, both at the cellular and physiological levels.

Managing and curtailing oxidative stress and inflammation is crucial to ward off their potential adverse effects on health and aging. A variety of strategies can be deployed towards this goal:

- Balanced Diet: A balanced diet rich in antioxidants is critical in fighting oxidative stress. Antioxidants, abundant in fruits, vegetables, nuts, seeds, and whole grains, can neutralize free radicals and limit their destructive effects. Certain foods, like fatty fish, berries, olive oil, and green tea, also exhibit anti-inflammatory properties.

- Regular Exercise: Physical activity can bolster the body's antioxidant defenses and curtail inflammation. Regular, moderate-intensity exercise can help maintain healthy weight, improve circulation, and enhance overall immune function.

- Stress Management: Chronic stress can aggravate both oxidative stress and inflammation. Techniques for managing stress, such as meditation, yoga, deep-breathing exercises, or other mindfulness practices, can help lower stress levels and lessen the inflammatory response.

- Adequate Sleep: Quality sleep is vital for various aspects of health, including the regulation of the immune response and oxidative stress. Chronic sleep deprivation can lead to heightened inflammation and oxidative stress.

- Avoidance of Toxins: Exposure to environmental toxins, including pollutants, cigarette smoke, and excessive alcohol, can contribute to oxidative stress and inflammation. Minimizing exposure to these toxins can help maintain a healthier balance.

- Medications or Supplements: In certain situations, medications or supplements may be used to help mitigate oxidative stress and inflammation. For instance, Non-Steroidal Anti-Inflammatory Drugs (NSAIDs) may be used to control inflammation, and antioxidant supplements may be beneficial in certain cases. However, these should always be used under the guidance of a healthcare provider, considering potential side effects and interactions.

Mushrooms and Longevity

For centuries, numerous societies have valued medicinal mushrooms for their beneficial health attributes. Modern scientific inquiries are now corroborating their historical usage by spotlighting their antioxidant and anti-inflammatory capabilities

Antioxidant Properties

Therapeutic mushrooms are laden with diverse compounds exhibiting antioxidant characteristics, including polysaccharides, phenolic and indolic substances, mycosteroids, fatty acids, carotenoids, vitamins (C, D, E, and B complex), and enzymes like superoxide dismutase and catalase.

Antioxidants work to counteract damaging free radicals within the body. As previously highlighted, free radicals can provoke oxidative stress, impairing cells, proteins, and DNA, and fostering aging and various diseases.

Several mushrooms are particularly recognized for their antioxidant prowess:

Reishi (Ganoderma lucidum): Reishi is abundant in antioxidants, including triterpenoids, polysaccharides, and phenolic compounds. It has been researched for its potential to combat oxidative stress and related diseases.

Chaga (Inonotus obliquus): Chaga boasts a wealth of antioxidants, especially melanin, a pigment bestowing Chaga its dark hue and exhibiting potent antioxidant attributes.

Anti-inflammatory Properties

Therapeutic mushrooms also encompass compounds capable of regulating the body's inflammatory response. Chronic inflammation can fuel numerous diseases, including heart disease, cancer, and neurodegenerative diseases.

Some noteworthy mushrooms with anti-inflammatory attributes include:

Cordyceps (Cordyceps sinensis and Cordyceps militaris): Cordyceps contain multiple compounds with anti-inflammatory properties, including cordycepin and polysaccharides. These compounds may inhibit the generation of pro-inflammatory cytokines, proteins that oversee and adjust inflammation.

Turkey Tail (Trametes versicolor): Turkey Tail features polysaccharides like polysaccharide-K (PSK) and polysaccharide peptide (PSP) that can regulate the immune system and diminish inflammation.

The Synergy of Antioxidant and Anti-inflammatory Effects

Medicinal mushrooms are highly esteemed for their potent antioxidant and anti-inflammatory properties, which work together to promote general health. This double-action capability makes them particularly beneficial in preventing and managing numerous diseases.

The antioxidants present in mushrooms serve to neutralize damaging free radicals within the body. These unstable molecules, if left unchecked, can inflict harm on cells and contribute to aging and conditions such as heart disease, cancer, and neurodegenerative disorders. By neutralizing these free radicals, mushroom antioxidants can safeguard our cells against this oxidative stress.

Furthermore, numerous medicinal mushrooms display anti-inflammatory qualities. They are loaded with compounds capable of modulating the body's immune reaction, thus mitigating excessive or prolonged inflammation. Chronic inflammation has been linked to an array of diseases, encompassing heart disease, diabetes, cancer, and neurodegenerative diseases like Alzheimer's.

The interplay of antioxidant and anti-inflammatory properties allows mushrooms to exert a robust protective effect against a broad spectrum of diseases. By diminishing both oxidative stress and inflammation, mushrooms contribute to maintaining the functional stability of cells and tissues, thereby promoting general health and wellness.

It is crucial to complement mushroom consumption with other healthy lifestyle habits to maximize benefits. An equilibrium diet abundant in diverse fruits, vegetables, lean proteins, healthy fats, and whole grains will provide a comprehensive range of nutrients vital for optimal health. Regular physical exercise is key for maintaining cardiovascular health, bolstering the immune system, managing weight, and enhancing mental wellbeing.

Telomeres and Aging

Telomeres, the little protective shields at the ends of our chromosomes akin to the plastic caps on shoelaces, are fundamental to our genetic health. Their primary role is to safeguard our genetic material as cells divide, assuring the flawless replication of DNA. But there's a hitch - with every cell division, these telomeres become shorter. Once they get too short, the cell either enters a state of dormancy, called senescence, or simply dies.

This reduction in telomere length is a natural process, and it's one of the ways our bodies show signs of aging. Because of this, the length of our telomeres can provide insights into our cellular age and overall health. Several age-related illnesses, including cardiovascular disease, diabetes, certain cancers, and dementia, have been linked to having shorter telomeres.

What's exciting is that initial research indicates that certain medicinal mushrooms, like Reishi (Ganoderma lucidum), might help guard against the shortening of telomeres. One study in the Journal of Ethnopharmacology in 2012 discovered that polysaccharides from Reishi mushrooms could delay telomere reduction in human lymphocytes, suggesting they might promote cell longevity.

Aging and the Role of Autophagy

Autophagy is a critical process within our cells where they break down and recycle their own components, akin to an internal recycling and waste management system. Through the elimination of damaged or unneeded cell components, autophagy helps maintain cellular balance and adapt to metabolic stress.

As we get older, autophagy becomes less efficient, leading to an accumulation of damaged cells and proteins, which can contribute to the onset of age-related diseases such as Alzheimer's, Parkinson's, and cancer.

Interestingly, specific compounds in mushrooms have been shown to stimulate autophagy. For instance, Cordycepin, found in the Cordyceps mushroom, has been shown in lab studies to initiate autophagy. A 2016 study in Oncotarget revealed that Cordycepin encouraged autophagy in human lung cancer cells, leading to their death.

Much of this research, it's important to note, has been conducted in lab or animal models, so we need more studies involving humans. However, these initial findings hint at another potential way that medicinal mushrooms could impact the aging process.

Chapter Six: Mushrooms and the Gut

The human gut microbiome is a complex and fascinating system that plays a significant role in health and disease. Here, we'll delve into understanding this vast ecosystem of microorganisms living in our digestive tract.

The term "gut microbiome," often interchangeably used with "gut flora," is used to describe the intricate network of trillions of microorganisms, primarily dwelling in our large intestine or colon. This ecosystem is amazingly diverse, hosting over a thousand identified bacterial species, alongside a myriad of viruses, fungi, protozoa, and other microbes.

Interestingly, we share a symbiotic relationship with these tiny inhabitants. They thrive in the warm, nutrient-rich environment of our gut, and in return, their activities greatly benefit us. These microbial partners are so crucial to our existence that some researchers view them as an additional organ in our bodies.

The composition of our gut microbiome is individual-specific and can be affected by various elements such as our genetic makeup, diet, age, medication usage (particularly antibiotics), stress levels, sleep habits, and so on. A healthy gut microbiome is marked by a diverse and balanced representation of different microbial species.

The gut microbiome undertakes several essential tasks that contribute significantly to our health and wellbeing:

- Food Digestion: Our gut microbiota plays an instrumental role in digesting the food we consume. They are particularly useful in breaking down dietary fibers and complex carbohydrates, substances our bodies struggle to digest independently. The microbes ferment these fibers and generate short-chain fatty acids like butyrate, propionate, and acetate. These fatty acids boast numerous health benefits, ranging from fueling our gut cells and managing our blood sugar levels to mitigating inflammation.

- Immune System Support: Nearly 70% of our immune system is based in our gut, and our gut microbiome significantly impacts its development and regulation. The gut microbes engage with immune cells, aiding in differentiating between harmful pathogens and innocuous or beneficial microbes. Moreover, they help modulate immune responses to avoid excessive reactions, which could otherwise trigger inflammation and autoimmune disorders.

- Gut Barrier Protection: Our gut microbiome also plays a role in maintaining the robustness of our gut barrier. A well-functioning gut barrier prevents potentially harmful substances from escaping the gut and infiltrating the bloodstream, a phenomenon commonly known as "leaky gut." Disruption in the gut microbiome could compromise this protective barrier, inciting inflammation and potentially contributing to a range of health issues, including inflammatory bowel disease, type 2 diabetes, and obesity.

Multiple elements can shape the composition and diversity of the gut microbiome, initiating right from the moment we're born:

- Mode of Delivery: Our inaugural interaction with microbes happens at the time of our birth. Infants born naturally are introduced to their mother's birth canal microbiota, which includes beneficial species like Bifidobacterium. However, babies born via a cesarean section encounter their first microbes from skin and the surroundings, leading to a distinct composition of their microbiome.

- Nutritional Intake: Our dietary choices play a substantial role in determining our gut microbiome's state. Consuming a varied diet abundant in whole foods, particularly fiber-loaded fruits, vegetables, legumes, and whole grains, fosters a more diverse and resilient gut microbiota. Dietary fiber acts like a prebiotic, feeding the beneficial gut bacteria. Conversely, a diet dominated by processed foods, sugars, and unhealthy fats can lead to a less diverse microbiome, potentially more vulnerable to dysbiosis (imbalance).

- Life Stage: Our gut microbiome continues to transform throughout our lifespan, from infancy to senior years. It tends to stabilize in adulthood, but diversity might decrease in elderly individuals, possibly leading to health concerns associated with aging.

- Pharmaceutical Interventions: Medicines, particularly antibiotics, can greatly alter the gut microbiome. Although antibiotics are sometimes necessary, they can annihilate beneficial bacteria along with the harmful ones, potentially causing both short-term and long-term shifts in the gut microbiome.

- Lifestyle Dynamics: Other lifestyle aspects, such as physical activity, sleep patterns, and stress levels, can also impact gut microbiota. Regular exercise and good sleep hygiene correlate with a healthier gut microbiome, while chronic stress might modify gut bacteria and weaken the gut barrier, potentially resulting in a leaky gut situation.

Growing recognition is being accorded to gut microbiota imbalances, referred to as dysbiosis, as contributing factors to various health problems:

- Digestive Disorders: Dysbiosis has been linked to several gastrointestinal complications, including irritable bowel syndrome (IBS), inflammatory bowel disease (IBD), and colorectal cancer.

- Metabolic Malfunctions: The gut microbiome might also have a say in metabolic disorders. For instance, specific gut bacteria can influence body weight and insulin sensitivity, potentially contributing to conditions like obesity and type 2 diabetes.

- Heart Disease: Certain gut bacteria are capable of transforming dietary elements into substances like trimethylamine N-oxide (TMAO), which might enhance heart disease risk.

- Mental Health: Emerging studies suggest a connection between the gut microbiome and mental health. This interaction, often referred to as the gut-brain axis, might have a role in mental health conditions such as anxiety, depression, and autism. Nonetheless, a significant portion of this research is still in preliminary stages, and more comprehensive studies are required to thoroughly comprehend these intricate relationships and explore potential strategies to manipulate the gut microbiome for treating these and other conditions.

Mushrooms Prebiotic Effects

As it turns out, mushrooms could function as potent prebiotics – a type of non-digestible fibers that nourish the beneficial gut bacteria.

Prebiotics, a class of indigestible dietary fiber, act as food for the good bacteria (probiotics) residing in our gut. Being resistant to human digestive enzymes, prebiotics transit almost untouched through the upper portion of our digestive system and undergo fermentation in the colon by the gut microbes. This process of fermentation gives rise to nutrients like short-chain fatty acids (SCFAs), which aid in maintaining a healthy gut bacterial population and fostering overall gut health.

Several varieties of prebiotics exist, including inulin, oligofructose, and galacto-oligosaccharides (GOS), commonly found in whole grains, bananas, onions, garlic, and leeks, among others.

Mushrooms, owing to their complex carbohydrate content, particularly polysaccharides, which resist digestion in the upper GI tract, serve as an excellent prebiotic source. These polysaccharides, such as beta-glucans, chitin, and others, provide nourishment for the good gut bacteria, encouraging their proliferation and activity.

The mycelium, the mushroom's network of thread-like roots, is exceptionally rich in these polysaccharides. For instance, the beta-glucan content of the mycelium has been observed to be higher than that in the fruiting body (the portion of the mushroom we typically consume, found above the ground).

The prebiotic influence of mushroom polysaccharides can impact gut health in numerous significant ways:

- Fostering Beneficial Bacteria: Mushroom-derived prebiotics, serving as a food source, can boost the growth and activity of beneficial gut bacteria, including Bifidobacterium and Lactobacillus species. These bacteria play a key part in various health-promoting functions, such as assisting digestion, producing vitamins, and suppressing the proliferation of harmful bacteria.

- Maintaining Gut Barrier Health: The fermentation of mushroom polysaccharides by gut bacteria yields short-chain fatty acids (SCFAs), including butyrate, propionate, and acetate. These SCFAs provide crucial energy to the cells lining the colon, supporting the maintenance of the gut barrier. This barrier prevents the seepage of harmful substances into the bloodstream, a phenomenon termed as "leaky gut".

- Modulating Immune Response: In addition to enhancing gut health, SCFAs and other bioactive compounds derived from the fermentation of mushroom polysaccharides can interact with the immune system. They play a significant role in managing immune responses and inflammation, exerting systemic effects that impact overall health and well-being.

In Practice

Incorporating mushrooms into your daily meals can be an effective way to enhance gut health, thanks to their prebiotic qualities. Both culinary and medicinal mushrooms like Shiitake, Reishi, Lion's Mane, and Turkey Tail are rich in polysaccharides, which nourish your gut microbes.

You can add mushrooms to a range of meals, from soups and salads to stir-fries, and even teas. This makes them easy to include in your diet. Thoroughly cooking mushrooms not only helps break down their cell walls, releasing the beneficial polysaccharides, but also minimizes potential anti-nutrients and toxins some mushrooms might contain.

Mushroom supplements, which usually contain the mycelium, can also offer these prebiotic benefits. These supplements come in different forms, like powders, capsules, and extracts, and provide a concentrated dose of mushroom polysaccharides, making them a convenient option.

Although mushrooms are generally considered safe for most people, high doses of mushroom supplements might lead to gastrointestinal discomfort in some individuals. Possible side effects include bloating, diarrhea, or constipation. To lessen the likelihood of these potential side effects, it's recommended to start with a small dosage and gradually increase as your body adjusts.

Certain mushrooms can interact with medications or have effects on blood clotting, blood sugar levels, and blood pressure. Therefore, those with existing health conditions should seek advice from a healthcare provider before starting any new supplement regimen.

Mushrooms and Digestive Disorders

An increasing volume of scientific study is investigating the possible benefits of mushrooms for handling digestive disorders. Various fungal species are being studied for their potential to enhance gut health and manage conditions like inflammatory bowel disease (IBD), irritable bowel syndrome (IBS), and other gastrointestinal (GI) issues.

Mushrooms and Inflammatory Bowel Disease

Inflammatory bowel disease (IBD) comprises disorders that involve long-term inflammation in the digestive tract, with Crohn's disease and ulcerative colitis being the most common. Current laboratory studies point towards the potential benefits of medicinal mushrooms for individuals dealing with IBD. Their anti-inflammatory and immune-system regulating properties show promise.

One specific mushroom, Agaricus blazei, has shown protective qualities against colitis in animal studies, mainly due to its polysaccharide content – long-chain carbohydrate molecules with immune-supporting properties. Preliminary research indicates that medicinal mushrooms might help control inflammatory responses in the gut, potentially alleviating IBD symptoms. However, human trials are limited, and more comprehensive research is needed to verify these findings and apply them in clinical settings.

Mushrooms and Irritable Bowel Syndrome (IBS)

Irritable bowel syndrome (IBS) is a functional disorder of the gastrointestinal (GI) tract, exhibiting symptoms such as abdominal discomfort, bloating, and changes in bowel habits. While there's limited research specifically examining the connection between mushrooms and IBS, the prebiotic potential of mushrooms – their capability to nourish beneficial gut bacteria – could theoretically aid those dealing with IBS. This is particularly pertinent for individuals with IBS subtypes where an imbalance of gut bacteria plays a significant role.

However, it's vital to remember that tolerance to dietary fiber can greatly vary among individuals with IBS, and for some, certain fiber types could exacerbate their symptoms. So, while the prebiotic attributes of mushrooms could potentially promote gut health in IBS, more specific research is required to fully understand this connection and its implications for treatment approaches.

Mushrooms and Gastric Ulcers

Certain medicinal mushrooms have demonstrated potential benefits for managing gastric ulcers in preliminary studies. Ganoderma lucidum, commonly known as Reishi mushroom, stands out in this context. Research has attributed potential anti-ulcer effects to various compounds within the Reishi mushroom. These compounds might inhibit the secretion of gastric acid, stimulate the production of protective mucus within the stomach, and exert anti-inflammatory effects.

These combined actions could potentially assist the healing process in gastric ulcers, helping to maintain the stomach's protective lining and reduce inflammation. Despite the potential demonstrated in these preliminary studies, it's crucial to undertake more comprehensive research, especially human clinical trials, to comprehend the full extent of Reishi and other mushrooms' therapeutic potential in managing gastric ulcers.

Incorporating Mushrooms into a Gut-Healthy Diet

Incorporating mushrooms into a gut-healthy diet can be a beneficial way to promote good digestive health. Mushrooms are rich in dietary fiber, including prebiotic types that can nourish your gut bacteria, and various compounds that may have anti-inflammatory and gut barrier-supporting effects. Here are some tips to incorporate mushrooms into your gut-healthy diet:

Mushroom Broth

The utilization of mushrooms in creating a nourishing stock presents an adaptable means of including them in your meals. This wholesome brew is produced by slowly cooking mushrooms along with other flavor-enhancing ingredients. The resulting broth, rich in umami taste, can either be enjoyed as a warming standalone beverage or used as a flavor-packed base for soups and stews. Apart from offering an excellent taste experience, the mushroom stock also carries the health advantages of the mushrooms used, which may include prebiotic fibers and an assortment of other beneficial substances. Furthermore, this method of preparation can make certain nutrients more readily absorbed in the body.

Dried Mushrooms

Desiccated mushrooms are a practical, extended shelf-life alternative to their fresh counterparts, especially when dealing with medicinal mushrooms not readily available in a fresh state. Once rehydrated, they can be employed in a manner similar to fresh mushrooms, being integrated into a variety of dishes from stir-fries to pasta.

Alternatively, desiccated mushrooms can be reduced to a fine dust and mixed into various foods and drinks. This mushroom dust can add flavor to soups, sauces, smoothies, or even teas, letting you gain the health benefits of mushrooms in a concentrated manner.

Fermented Mushroom Product

Fermentation, a process that not only preserves food but also boosts its nutritional worth, can be utilized with mushrooms. Products such as mushroom tempeh or certain mushroom teas undergo fermentation, yielding products that combine the benefits of mushrooms and the process of fermentation. Fermented foods are a significant source of probiotics - friendly bacteria that support a healthy gut microbiome. Consequently, fermented mushroom products can contribute to your well-being by offering both the prebiotic benefits of mushrooms and the probiotic benefits of fermentation.

The Importance of Variety

Just as diversity is crucial in many nutritional aspects, the same holds true for mushrooms. Consuming an assortment of mushrooms ensures you're receiving a wide spectrum of prebiotics and other health-promoting compounds, each with their distinct health properties. From everyday culinary types like button mushrooms and shiitake to medicinal ones like Reishi and Lion's Mane, there's a vast array of mushrooms to discover. Each species offers different tastes and nutritional profiles, so don't be afraid to experiment and discover your personal favorites. By incorporating a selection of these fungi in your diet, you'll be maximizing their potential benefits to your health.

Chapter Seven: Mushrooms and Heart Health

Cardiovascular disorders, also known as heart diseases, is an umbrella term that includes various ailments impacting the heart and blood vessels. Frequent examples of heart diseases are coronary artery disease, heart failure, and arrhythmias. It's vital to comprehend the causes and risk elements for heart diseases for their prevention and control.

Causes of Heart Disease

The term heart disease covers an array of conditions affecting the heart. Let's delve deeper into some of the causes associated with different types of heart diseases:

Coronary Artery Disease (CAD): The most prevalent form of heart disease, CAD, is often triggered by atherosclerosis, a situation in which fatty deposits (plaque) accumulate in the coronary arteries, the vessels that supply the heart muscle with oxygen and nutrients. Over time, this plaque, which hardens and narrows the arteries, can restrict the heart's blood supply, possibly leading to chest discomfort (angina) or a heart attack. Aspects contributing to plaque formation include elevated cholesterol levels, smoking, and inflammation.

Heart Failure: Also termed congestive heart failure, this ailment arises when the heart is incapable of pumping sufficient blood to cater to the body's requirements. Heart failure often follows damage to the heart muscle, which can result from a heart attack, high blood pressure, or other heart conditions. It can also occur due to conditions that overstrain the heart, such as obesity, thyroid disease, or kidney disease.

Arrhythmias: Arrhythmias denote irregular heart rhythms, which can be too rapid, too slow, or erratic. Arrhythmias can be caused by numerous factors, including heart disease, scarring of the heart from a prior heart attack, hypertension, certain medications, and imbalances of electrolytes in the body.

Risk Factors

Several factors can heighten the probability of developing heart disease:

Age: With advancing age, the risk of heart disease tends to rise, largely attributable to the gradual wear and tear of the cardiovascular system over time.

Sex: Males tend to be at a greater risk of heart disease, although the risk for females significantly increases after menopause.

Family History: If a direct relative (a parent or sibling) has suffered from heart disease, particularly at a young age, the risk of developing the condition is greater.

Smoking: Smoking harms the lining of the blood vessels, facilitating the accumulation of plaque and increasing the risk of atherosclerosis and heart disease.

Diet: A diet high in saturated fats, trans fats, cholesterol, and salt can aid in the development of heart disease by escalating blood pressure, leading to weight gain, and raising cholesterol levels.

Physical Inactivity: A sedentary lifestyle can contribute to heart disease by encouraging obesity, hypertension, and high cholesterol, among other risk factors.

Obesity: Being overweight, particularly carrying surplus weight around the abdomen, heightens the strain on the heart and raises the risk of developing heart disease.

High Blood Pressure (Hypertension): Chronic hypertension can overtax the heart and injure the blood vessels, making them more prone to plaque accumulation.

High Cholesterol: Elevated levels of LDL cholesterol (the "bad" cholesterol) or low levels of HDL cholesterol (the "good" cholesterol) can promote atherosclerosis, thereby increasing the risk of heart disease.

Diabetes: Particularly when poorly controlled, diabetes significantly increases the risk of heart disease. High blood sugar levels can injure blood vessels and facilitate plaque formation.

Chronic Stress or Depression: Psychological elements such as persistent stress or depression can aid in the development of heart disease, likely through intricate mechanisms involving the nervous system, immune system, and inflammation.

Preventing heart disease involves managing these risk factors, which often includes making lifestyle changes such as eating a heart-healthy diet, exercising regularly, not smoking, managing stress, and controlling conditions like high blood pressure and diabetes. Regular check-ups with a healthcare provider can also help detect any early signs of heart disease. Always consult with a healthcare provider for personalized advice on preventing and managing heart disease.

Mushrooms in Heart Health

Mushrooms are nutritional powerhouses, packed with dietary fiber, vitamins, and minerals, as well as unique health-promoting compounds that could support heart health. Let's explore the scientific findings:

Reducing Cholesterol Levels

Some types of mushrooms, like Shiitake, are known to contain substances such as eritadenine and beta-glucans, which have demonstrated abilities to decrease levels of low-density lipoprotein (LDL), or the so-called "bad" cholesterol. LDL cholesterol is infamous for its propensity to gather in blood vessel walls, leading to plaque buildup, a condition referred to as atherosclerosis. Consequently, high LDL cholesterol levels may heighten the risk of heart diseases. The cholesterol-reducing properties in mushrooms function differently. It's believed that eritadenine aids in expelling cholesterol from the body, while beta-glucans hinder cholesterol absorption in the digestive tract.

Regulating Blood Pressure

Some mushrooms, like Maitake and Reishi, are rich in natural compounds that could aid in blood pressure regulation. Hypertension or high blood pressure can overstrain the heart and damage blood vessels, thereby enhancing the risk of heart diseases. It's thought that mushrooms' blood pressure-lowering effects originate from compounds like ganoderic acids (found in Reishi) and polysaccharides (found in Maitake). These compounds can block an enzyme that narrows blood vessels, thus promoting the relaxation and dilation of these vessels.

Assisting Weight Management

Mushrooms can also assist in weight management, which is vital for maintaining heart health. They are low in calories, abundant in water, and filled with fiber, which can help regulate appetite and decrease total caloric consumption. Furthermore, mushrooms are flavorful and adaptable, making them an excellent replacement for high-calorie ingredients in numerous recipes. By facilitating weight management, mushrooms could aid in averting obesity, a significant heart disease risk factor.

Vitamin D Content

Certain mushrooms, especially those exposed to ultraviolet (UV) light, are a valuable source of vitamin D from the plant kingdom. This nutrient is crucial for heart health. Lack of vitamin D has been associated with an increased risk of heart diseases, given that the vitamin plays a key role in controlling blood pressure, managing inflammation, and overseeing glucose metabolism, among other processes. Although few foods naturally carry vitamin D, mushrooms exposed to UV light can produce this nutrient when they come into contact with sunlight, similar to human skin.

Tips for Including Mushrooms in a Heart-Healthy Diet

With their hearty texture and savory, umami taste, mushrooms serve as an excellent meat replacement in a variety of meals, from burgers and sautés to casseroles and pasta sauces. This substitution can be advantageous for cardiovascular health, as decreasing meat intake, especially red and processed meats, can reduce the consumption of saturated fats and cholesterol, both of which are linked to a higher risk of heart disease. Furthermore, utilizing mushrooms in place of meat can augment your intake of heart-beneficial nutrients like fiber, vitamins, and antioxidants.

Incorporating raw or lightly cooked mushrooms into salads and sautés not only enriches the flavor and texture of these dishes but also boosts their nutritional value. Mushrooms provide vital nutrients, including B vitamins, selenium, and potassium, all of which are involved in maintaining heart health. Additionally, if you're cutting back on meat, mushrooms can lend a satisfying heartiness to these meals.

A broth made from simmering mushrooms with a selection of herbs and spices creates a robust and tasty foundation for soups and stews. This method is not only a cozy and soothing way to relish mushrooms during chillier seasons, but it's also a smart strategy to draw out and consume their health-promoting compounds. Hence, integrating mushroom-based broths and soups into your diet can enhance heart health.

Grilling or roasting mushrooms can amplify their inherent, earthy tastes, making them an enjoyable side dish or a savory addition to various recipes, from pizzas and pastas to grain bowls and roasted vegetables. The dry heat from grilling or roasting helps decrease the water content in mushrooms, which can enhance their flavor and potentially their nutrient concentration as well.

Mushroom powders, prepared from dried and pulverized mushrooms, offer a handy way to integrate the health advantages of mushrooms into your diet. They can be effortlessly blended into smoothies, combined into sauces, dusted over soups, or even incorporated into baked goods. This allows you to harness the benefits of mushrooms without significantly changing the texture of your dishes, which is particularly useful if you wish to incorporate medicinal mushroom varieties that aren't commonly used in culinary preparation.

Chapter Eight: Mushrooms and Cancer

Cancer refers to a diverse set of diseases marked by the uncontrolled multiplication and migration of irregular cells. Over 100 kinds of cancer exist, which include breast, skin, lung, colon, prostate cancer, and lymphoma. Cancer's origin can be traced back to an assortment of factors such as lifestyle, environmental influences, and certain genetic alterations that transpire over a person's lifetime.

Causes and Risk Elements

Cancer emerges when the body's standard control mechanisms cease to function properly. Old cells do not perish, instead they amass to form a mass, known as a tumor. Not all tumors are cancerous; benign tumors do not infiltrate other body parts and are not fatal. Malignant tumors, however, can invade and damage nearby tissues. Here are some notable causes and risk factors:

Genetics: It is projected that 5-10% of all cancers are directly due to inherited genetic flaws, or mutations transmitted from one generation to the next. Certain types of cancers, like breast, ovarian, colorectal, and prostate cancer, often have a genetic association. Yet, most cancers result from genetic changes that occur throughout a person's lifetime as a consequence of aging and exposure to environmental elements such as tobacco smoke and radiation.

Lifestyle: Lifestyle elements include habits that individuals adopt as part of their life. These encompass unhealthy diet, sedentary lifestyle, and excessive alcohol intake. Tobacco use, for instance, is the most substantial risk factor for cancer and accounts for approximately 22% of global cancer deaths. Likewise, excessive alcohol consumption is a major risk factor for various cancers, including those of the mouth, esophagus, throat, liver, and breast.

Environment: The surroundings in which we reside and work can also amplify the risk of developing specific types of cancer. Contact with certain substances has been associated with particular types of cancer. These substances are called carcinogens. For instance, inhaling asbestos fibers can lead to lung diseases, including lung cancer and mesothelioma. Similarly, exposure to certain types of radiation, such as ultraviolet rays and ionizing radiation, can considerably heighten the risk of skin cancer and leukemia, respectively.

Chronic Inflammation: Chronic inflammation caused by infections or inflammatory conditions can contribute to cancer development. For instance, individuals with chronic inflammatory bowel diseases, like Crohn's disease or ulcerative colitis, have a heightened risk of colon cancer. Likewise, individuals with chronic viral infections like hepatitis B and C have an increased risk of developing liver cancer.

Symptoms

Cancer symptoms depend on its location, size, and its impact on the organs or tissues. If cancer has spread (metastasized), signs or symptoms may appear in various body parts. The following are some general signs and symptoms:

Fatigue: Inexplicable and constant fatigue might indicate the body is combating cancerous cells or there's a presence of a large tumor. This fatigue is not alleviated by rest and can be an early cancer sign.

Weight Loss: Unexplained weight loss is often one of the earliest discernible symptoms of cancers of the pancreas, stomach, esophagus, or lung.

Pain: Constant or worsening pain is usually a symptom of various types of cancer. This can be due to a tumor pressing on nerves, bones, or organs. The pain can occur in the early stages of some cancers, like testicular or bone cancers.

Skin Changes: Certain cancers can cause visible skin changes, such as darker looking skin (hyperpigmentation), yellowish skin and eyes (jaundice), reddened skin (erythema), itching (pruritus), and excessive hair growth.

Changes in Bowel or Bladder Function: Prolonged constipation, diarrhea, or a change in stool size could signal colon cancer. Pain during urination, blood in urine, or a change in bladder function could be related to bladder or prostate cancer.

Unusual Bleeding: Abnormal bleeding can occur in early or advanced cancer. Blood in the stool could signal colon or rectal cancer. Coughing up blood may hint at lung cancer.

Blood in the urine could mean bladder or kidney cancer. Unusual vaginal bleeding could suggest cervical or endometrial cancer.

Persistent Cough or Difficulty Swallowing: A persistent cough could hint at lung cancer. Trouble swallowing is often associated with esophageal or throat cancer.

Diagnosis

The process of diagnosing cancer involves a sequence of steps that confirm the existence of cancer and establish the specific variety, site, and stage of the disease. The process generally initiates with a consultation with a medical professional following the recognition of symptoms, with the steps often including:

Physical Examination: The healthcare provider carries out a physical examination to look for any irregularities. They might search for physical indications of cancer, like lumps, changes in skin, or an organ's enlargement.

Medical History Review: The healthcare provider will assemble a thorough personal and family medical history. This can comprise information about symptoms, risk factors, previous illnesses, treatments, and more. The collected medical history can hint at the potential condition and inform further testing.

Imaging Procedures: Imaging procedures generate images of internal body sections, assisting the healthcare provider in identifying if a tumor exists. These tests can include X-rays, CT scans, MRI scans, PET scans, and ultrasound.

Laboratory Assessments: Lab assessments, including blood and urine tests, can aid in identifying irregularities that might suggest cancer. For instance, a complete blood count (CBC) test is commonly used because it can assess overall health and spot disorders like anemia or infection.

Biopsy: In many instances, the healthcare provider may request a biopsy, which requires the removal of a small tissue sample for microscopic examination. The cells in the sample are evaluated to ascertain if they are cancerous, the cancer type, and the cancer grade (how abnormal the cells appear and how swiftly the cancer is expected to grow and spread).

Therapy Methods

Cancer therapy may involve a single approach or a combination of therapies. The required treatment type depends on the cancer type, stage, and location, as well as the person's overall health. Here are some common treatment methods:

Surgical Treatment: Surgical treatment is frequently utilized to diagnose, stage, and treat cancer, and to manage specific cancer-related symptoms. The surgeon aims to excise the entire tumor, or as much as possible. In some scenarios, it might be used in combination with other treatments like chemotherapy or radiation therapy.

Radiation Therapy: Radiation therapy is a form of cancer treatment that employs beams of intense energy to exterminate cancer cells. The radiation might come from a machine outside the body (external-beam radiation therapy), or from radioactive material placed in the body near cancer cells (internal radiation therapy or brachytherapy).

Chemotherapy: Chemotherapy is a form of cancer treatment that employs drugs to eliminate cancer cells. It functions by halting or slowing the proliferation of cancer cells, which grow and divide swiftly. It can be administered in many ways, including pill form or injection.

Immunotherapy: Immunotherapy is a form of cancer treatment that aids your immune system in fighting cancer. The body's immune system assists in fighting infections and other diseases. In some types of immunotherapy, treatments boost your immune system to work better against cancer. In others, they introduce engineered immune system proteins to combat cancer cells.

Targeted Therapy: Targeted therapy is a form of cancer treatment that employs drugs or other substances to identify and assault cancer cells while causing minimal damage to healthy cells. These therapies target the cancer's specific genes, proteins, or the tissue environment contributing to cancer growth and survival.

Hormone Therapy: Hormone therapy is a treatment that slows or stops the growth of breast and prostate cancers that rely on hormones to grow. Hormone therapy is often utilized alongside other cancer treatments.

Stem Cell Transplantation: Stem cell transplantation, also known as a bone marrow transplant, is a procedure that introduces healthy blood-forming stem cells into the body.

It's used to replace bone marrow that's been destroyed by cancer or destroyed by high doses of chemotherapy or radiation therapy used to treat the cancer. Stem cell transplants are most often used in the treatment of leukemias and lymphomas.

Bioactive Compounds and Anti-cancer Properties of Mushrooms

Mushrooms are plentiful in health-boosting compounds that have been researched for their possible anti-cancer traits. These elements operate in various ways, such as hindering the proliferation of cancer cells, instigating the self-destruction of cancer cells (apoptosis), and boosting the body's immune response towards cancer cells. The following are some of the health-boosting compounds in mushrooms notable for their possible anti-cancer characteristics:

Polysaccharides

Complex carbohydrates, particularly beta-glucans, are intricate sugars found abundantly in various types of mushrooms. They have garnered scientific interest due to their health-promoting activities, which include immune system modulation and anti-cancer effects.

Beta-glucans invigorate the immune system by activating different immune cells like macrophages, natural killer cells, and T cells, and by boosting the production of immune mediators. This can result in an enhanced immune response against cancer cells.

An example of a mushroom-derived complex carbohydrate with anti-cancer properties is lentinan, a beta-glucan found in Shiitake mushrooms. Lentinan doesn't directly destroy cancer cells; instead, it enhances the immune system, which can help the body combat cancer. In Japan, lentinan is used as an adjunct in the treatment of stomach cancer, meaning it's employed along with standard cancer treatments to improve their efficacy.

Terpenoids

Organic compounds, specifically terpenoids, are a large and diverse collection of naturally occurring organic chemicals derived from five-carbon isoprene units. They are found in many types of organisms, including mushrooms. In mushrooms like Reishi (Ganoderma lucidum), terpenoids have demonstrated noteworthy anti-cancer properties.

Notably, some mushroom-derived terpenoids have demonstrated the capability to inhibit the proliferation of cancer cells, induce apoptosis (a process of programmed cell destruction that occurs when cells are damaged or under stress), and prevent metastasis (the migration of cancer cells from the primary site to other parts of the body). They achieve this by influencing various cellular pathways that regulate cell survival and growth.

Lectins

Proteins, specifically lectins, are a type of protein found in a wide array of organisms, including mushrooms. They have the capability to bind to specific carbohydrate structures, particularly those on cell surfaces. This binding ability can have various biological effects.

Lectins derived from mushrooms have been found to exhibit anti-cancer properties. For instance, they can inhibit the growth and proliferation of cancer cells, instigate apoptosis, and even prevent the adhesion and migration of cancer cells, which are key steps in metastasis. However, the precise mechanisms through which these lectins exercise their anti-cancer effects are still being explored. Like with other health-boosting compounds, these findings need to be confirmed and further examined in clinical trials.

Fungal Immunomodulatory Proteins

Proteins Influencing Immune Responses from Fungi (PIRFs) are a category of proteins originating from mushrooms that possess the capability to modify the body's immune reactions. Instances of such proteins have been detected in several mushroom types, including the edible Flammulina velutipes, more commonly known as enoki mushroom.

Studies suggest that PIRFs can demonstrate a variety of biological influences, encompassing anti-inflammatory, anti-allergic, and anti-cancer activities. Regarding cancer, PIRFs are believed to function by bolstering the activity of the immune system. For instance, they might enhance the cytotoxic efficiency of natural killer cells (cells capable of eliminating cancer cells) and stimulate the production of cytokines (molecules that enable communication among immune cells).

These immune-boosting influences of PIRFs can assist the body in more effectively identifying and destroying cancer cells, thereby decelerating cancer progression and improving survival chances. However, additional studies are required to thoroughly comprehend the potential of PIRFs as anti-cancer agents, inclusive of clinical trials involving humans.

Ergosterol derivatives

Ergosterol is a sterol present in the cell membranes of fungi, including mushrooms, and performs a role analogous to that of cholesterol in animal cells. When mushrooms that contain ergosterol are exposed to ultraviolet light, ergosterol is converted into ergocalciferol, also referred to as vitamin D2.

Ergosterol peroxide is an oxidized derivative of ergosterol. Research indicates that ergosterol peroxide possesses several biological activities, including anti-inflammatory, antioxidant, and anti-cancer activities. In relation to cancer, studies suggest that ergosterol peroxide can hinder the proliferation of cancer cells and incite apoptosis, a form of programmed cell death. It's believed to achieve this by interfering with various cellular pathways that control cell growth and survival.

In spite of promising results from laboratory studies, further research is necessary to fully comprehend how ergosterol and its derivatives might be utilized in the prevention or treatment of cancer. This includes clinical trials to assess their efficacy and safety in humans.

Mushrooms and Cancer-Preventative Lifestyle

Embedding an assortment of mushrooms into your dietary habits can be a method to capitalize on the multitude of nutrients and bioactive substances offered by different mushroom species. Types of mushrooms such as Shiitake, Maitake, Reishi, and Oyster are acknowledged for their potential health-enhancing qualities, encompassing immune-boosting attributes and the existence of components linked with anti-cancer activities. Consuming a mix of mushrooms ensures you benefit from a wider scope of these health-supporting substances. For instance, you might include Shiitake mushrooms in a stir-fry, employ Maitake mushrooms in a soup, or relish a Reishi mushroom tea.

Cooking Methods

Mushrooms exhibit versatility and can be incorporated into the diet through various means. They can be enjoyed raw in salads, sautéed and incorporated into meals, roasted for a profound, savory taste, grilled for a smoky flavor, or added to soups and stews for a nutrient enhancement. However, while certain mushrooms can be consumed raw, it's crucial to consider that cooking them can assist in breaking down potentially damaging compounds, improve digestibility, and might even enhance their nutritional profile. Some compounds in mushrooms become more bioavailable (simpler for your body to absorb and utilize) post-cooking. As such, it's generally advisable to cook mushrooms prior to consumption.

Diversify Your Diet

Despite the potential health advantages of mushrooms, it's vital to recall that they constitute just one segment of a balanced, nutritious diet. A diet that could aid in preventing cancer typically comprises high quantities of fruits, vegetables, whole grains, lean proteins, and healthy fats, and low quantities of processed foods, sugary beverages, and red and processed meats. Combining mushrooms with a variety of these other nutritious foods can optimize your intake of an extensive range of nutrients and plant compounds beneficial for comprehensive health. For instance, you might have a salad with raw vegetables and grilled mushrooms, a whole grain pasta dish with sautéed mushrooms and lean chicken, or a stir-fry with a variety of vegetables and sliced Shiitake mushrooms.

Chapter Nine: Practical Guide to Consuming Medicinal Mushrooms

Mushrooms form a key segment of our food intake, with an extensive historical background in traditional healthcare practices and a noteworthy nutritional composition. However, the argument over whether it's more beneficial to ingest mushrooms in their raw state or post-cooking remains a topic of discussion, with each approach offering its own merits and potential pitfalls.

Eating mushrooms in their natural, uncooked form helps to preserve some nutrients, like vitamin C, that may lessen when subjected to heat during cooking. Additionally, certain enzymes found in fresh mushrooms can possibly aid in digestion and enhance the absorption of nutritional elements.

Nevertheless, the cellular composition of raw mushrooms can be rather sturdy, potentially making it more difficult for our bodies to digest and take advantage of the nutrients they house. Consuming raw mushrooms also has some possible drawbacks. For instance, some mushroom varieties harbor minute amounts of compounds that could prove detrimental. Button mushrooms, specifically, contain a compound dubbed agaritine, recognized as a potential carcinogen, although the risk associated with its consumption is viewed as relatively low. This compound's presence notably diminishes when these mushrooms are subjected to cooking.

Cooking mushrooms not only aids in ensuring their safety for consumption but also assists in unlocking their nutrient content, making it more readily accessible and easier for your body to assimilate. The heat from cooking aids in dismantling the cell walls of mushrooms, primarily composed of chitin, a substance that our digestive systems might find challenging to break down. This procedure effectively frees the beneficial compounds lodged within these cell walls, which incorporate vitamins, minerals, and other bioactive substances.

One specific nutrient, beta-glucans, attains enhanced bioavailability through the cooking process. Beta-glucans are a kind of soluble fiber detected in mushrooms, hailed for their immune-enhancement properties and potential anti-cancer activity. Moreover, the antioxidant content in mushrooms, specifically a compound known as ergothioneine, either remains intact or may even amplify through cooking, offering additional health-enhancing benefits. This antioxidant is recognized for its potential function in curbing inflammation and shielding cells from oxidative damage, a factor contributing to aging and disease progression.

Hence, while eating raw mushrooms might hold certain benefits, cooking them could potentially offer superior nutritional advantages and safety assurance.

Cooking Methods

The selected approach to preparing mushrooms can significantly affect the nutrient profile and their bioavailability. Here's a deeper look into each method:

Grilling and Heating in a Microwave: Grilling and using a microwave are some of the most efficient techniques for preserving a high level of antioxidant activity in mushrooms. These methods subject mushrooms to intense heat for a relatively brief duration, helping to maintain the stability of their nutrients. Additionally, microwaving and barbecuing do not involve water, which could dilute soluble nutrients. Barbecuing, specifically, can boost the taste of mushrooms, imparting them with a delicious, lightly charred flavor.

Simmering: Simmering mushrooms could lead to a substantial depletion of valuable nutrients. This is due to the fact that many compounds found in mushrooms are soluble in water, which means they can dissolve into the water during the simmering process. These could include proteins, antioxidants, and vitamins such as the vitamin B group and vitamin C. If you decide to simmer mushrooms, it would be advantageous to use the cooking water in broths, soups, or sauces to ensure these nutrients aren't wasted.

Sautéing: Sautéing mushrooms in a small quantity of healthy fats, like avocado oil or olive oil, can facilitate the absorption of fat-soluble nutrients present in mushrooms. These encompass ergosterol, a compound that can transform into vitamin D when subjected to UV light. Moreover, the high temperatures and rapid cooking duration in pan-frying can help maintain a considerable portion of the mushrooms' nutrients, while imparting a delightful texture and intensified flavor.

Baking: Baking is a dry heat preparation method that can preserve a significant amount of the nutrients found in mushrooms. It's a particularly appropriate method for handling larger or thicker mushroom types, like Portobello mushrooms. Roasting can enhance the flavor of mushrooms by triggering a process known as the Maillard reaction, which results in a tasty browning effect. Just remember to avoid exposing them to extremely high temperatures and extending the roasting times excessively, as these could lead to nutrient loss.

Supplements vs Whole Mushrooms

While whole, fresh mushrooms are a staple in many kitchens, medicinal mushroom supplements have also become increasingly popular. Both forms offer the potential benefits of mushrooms, but there are some important differences to understand.

Whole Mushrooms

Consuming whole fungi, either in fresh or dried form, enables you to take advantage of the full spectrum of their nutrients, encompassing dietary fiber, a variety of vitamins and minerals, and numerous bioactive components such as beta-glucans and antioxidants. Moreover, fungi are a low-calorie food source that can enhance the taste and texture of a multitude of meals.

Nevertheless, the bioavailability of certain components, specifically beta-glucans, may be reduced in uncooked fungi due to their intricate cellular structure. As addressed in the previous section, cooking processes can assist in breaking down these cellular walls and enhancing bioavailability. Additionally, some fungi may not be easily accessible in local supermarkets, and various types of therapeutic fungi are not traditionally incorporated in culinary practices.

Mushroom Supplements

Nutraceuticals derived from fungi, which are available as powders, capsules, or liquid extracts, are prepared from either the mycelium (the root-like formation of fungi) cultivated on grains or the fruiting part of the fungi itself. These nutraceuticals are typically employed to deliver a potent dosage of particular compounds, such as beta-glucans.

Nutraceuticals offer a more straightforward way to integrate medicinal fungi into your dietary regimen, especially if you find the taste of fungi unpalatable, or if you're seeking the advantages of specific types of fungi that are not readily available or not traditionally used in culinary practices.

Nonetheless, the standard of fungi-based nutraceuticals can differ greatly. Some products may not feature the types or amounts of compounds as stated on the packaging. It's essential to purchase nutraceuticals from trusted manufacturers who implement stringent quality control procedures.

Furthermore, while nutraceuticals can deliver potent quantities of particular compounds, they may not provide the diverse array of nutrients found in whole fungi.

Potential Side Effects

Although fungi have been part of human diets for ages and are generally deemed harmless, it's essential to stay informed about potential side effects and interactions, especially when they are consumed in large quantities or as dietary supplements.

Allergic Reactions: Fungi are savored by many for their unique flavor and potential health benefits. However, in some cases, they may trigger allergic responses. Such reactions are instigated by the immune system's reaction to specific proteins or other substances present in fungi. Mild symptoms might encompass skin reactions like itchiness, inflammation, or hives. Occasionally, the reaction can be severe, leading to respiratory difficulties, dizziness, or anaphylaxis, a potentially fatal allergic reaction that necessitates immediate medical intervention. Individuals with known allergies to fungi should refrain from consuming them. Even if you haven't had a prior reaction to fungi, it's crucial to seek immediate medical assistance if you exhibit any allergic reaction symptoms after consuming them.

Digestive Discomfort: Some individuals might experience digestive unease after consuming fungi, particularly if they aren't accustomed to them or if they are consumed raw. This might manifest as bloating, gas, or diarrhea. The cell walls of fungi comprise chitin, a complex carbohydrate that is not easily metabolized by the human digestive system. This might trigger digestive discomfort, especially when fungi are consumed in large volumes. Cooking can assist in breaking down these cell walls and possibly make fungi easier to digest.

Toxicity: While numerous types of fungi are edible and potentially health-boosting, others are poisonous and can cause serious sickness or even be lethal if ingested. Symptoms of fungi poisoning can fluctuate extensively depending on the type of fungi consumed, but might encompass vomiting, diarrhea, abdominal discomfort, hallucinations, convulsions, and liver damage. To circumvent the risk of fungi poisoning, it is imperative to consume only fungi that have been correctly identified as safe. This entails buying fungi from a trustworthy source or, if foraging, being absolutely certain of the fungi's identity. If there's any doubt, it's always safer to refrain from consuming them.

Drug Interactions: Certain substances in fungi can interact with specific drugs, potentially affecting their efficacy or causing unwanted effects. For example, specific types of therapeutic fungi are known to possess blood-thinning (anticoagulant) properties. If you're taking blood-thinning drugs, consuming these fungi could potentially escalate the risk of bleeding. Similarly, some fungi can affect blood sugar levels and might interfere with the efficacy of diabetes drugs. If you're on medication and contemplating incorporating therapeutic fungi or fungi supplements into your dietary regimen, it's crucial to consult with a healthcare professional first to evade potential interactions.

Immune Response: Fungi are recognized for their immunomodulatory attributes, chiefly due to their high concentration of polysaccharides like beta-glucans. These compounds can invigorate the immune system, boosting its capability to ward off infections and illnesses. However, in individuals diagnosed with autoimmune disorders, where the immune system erroneously attacks the body's own cells, this immune stimulation could potentially intensify symptoms or trigger episodes. While investigations in this domain are still in the initial stages, anyone with an autoimmune disorder should have a dialogue with their healthcare provider before introducing high quantities of fungi or fungi supplements into their dietary regimen.

Special Population: Certain demographic groups might need to exercise caution when consuming fungi or fungi supplements. For instance, women who are pregnant or nursing should always have a conversation with a healthcare provider before significantly escalating their consumption of fungi or initiating any fungi supplement, as the safety of numerous fungi compounds for these groups has not been extensively researched. Similarly, children's bodies can respond differently to substances than adults', and thus parents should converse with a pediatrician before introducing fungi supplements into a child's dietary regimen. Individuals suffering from severe or chronic health issues should also discuss any dietary modifications or new supplement routines with their healthcare provider, due to the potential for interactions or adverse effects.

Simple and Nutritious Mushroom Recipes

Here are a few simple and nutritious recipes that incorporate mushrooms, highlighting their versatility in the kitchen.

Mushroom Soup

Ingredients

- 1 lb fresh mushrooms (shiitake, cremini, or a mix)

- 1 medium onion, chopped

- 2 cloves garlic, minced

- 4 cups vegetable broth

- Salt and pepper to taste

- Fresh herbs (thyme, parsley, or dill), for garnish

Procedure

- Clean the mushrooms and slice them thinly.

- In a large pot, sauté the onions in a bit of olive oil until translucent.

- Add the garlic and mushrooms, and cook until the mushrooms have released their liquid.

- Add the vegetable broth, bring to a boil, then lower the heat and let it simmer for about 20 minutes.

- Blend half of the soup to create a creamy texture while maintaining some mushroom pieces for texture, or blend fully if you prefer a smooth soup.

- Season with salt and pepper, and garnish with fresh herbs before serving.

Stir-fried Mushrooms and Veggies

Ingredients:

- 1 lb fresh mushrooms (like oyster or shiitake)

- 2 bell peppers, sliced

- 1 medium onion, sliced

- 2 cloves garlic, minced

- 2 tbsp low-sodium soy sauce or tamari

- 1 tbsp sesame oil

Procedure:

- Clean the mushrooms and cut them into pieces.

- Heat the sesame oil in a pan, add the onions and garlic, and sauté until the onions are translucent.

- Add the mushrooms and peppers, and stir-fry for about 5-7 minutes, until the vegetables are tender.

- Add the soy sauce, stir well to combine, and cook for another minute.

- Serve hot, ideally over brown rice or quinoa.

Grilled Portobello Mushroom Caps:

Ingredients:

- 4 large Portobello mushrooms

- 2 tbsp olive oil

- 1 tbsp balsamic vinegar

- 1 clove garlic, minced

- Salt and pepper to taste

- Fresh herbs (like rosemary or thyme)

Procedure:

- Clean the mushrooms and remove the stems.

- In a bowl, mix the olive oil, balsamic vinegar, garlic, salt, and pepper.

- Brush the mushroom caps with this mixture, making sure to coat them well.

- Grill the mushrooms for about 5-7 minutes on each side, until they are tender and well-cooked.

- Garnish with fresh herbs before serving.

Mushroom and Spinach Frittata

Ingredients:

- 8 eggs

- 1 lb fresh mushrooms (like cremini or white)

- 2 cups fresh spinach

- 1 medium onion, chopped

- 2 cloves garlic, minced

- Salt and pepper to taste

- 1/2 cup grated cheese (optional)

Procedure:

- Preheat your oven to 350°F (175°C).

- Clean the mushrooms and slice them thinly.

- In a large, oven-safe pan, sauté the onions and garlic in a bit of olive oil until the onions are translucent.

- Add the mushrooms and cook until they've released their liquid. Then, add the spinach and cook until wilted.

- In a separate bowl, whisk the eggs and season with salt and pepper. Pour the egg mixture over the vegetables in the pan.

- If using cheese, sprinkle it on top.

- Bake in the preheated oven for about 20-25 minutes, until the eggs are set.

Mushroom and Lentil Stew

Ingredients:

- 1 lb fresh mushrooms (like shiitake or Portobello)

- 1 cup lentils

- 1 large carrot, chopped

- 1 medium onion, chopped

- 2 cloves garlic, minced

- 4 cups vegetable broth

- 1 tsp dried thyme

- Salt and pepper to taste

- Fresh parsley, for garnish

Procedure:

- Clean the mushrooms and cut them into pieces.

- In a large pot, sauté the onions and garlic in a bit of olive oil until the onions are translucent.

- Add the mushrooms, carrot, lentils, and thyme, and stir well to combine.

- Add the vegetable broth, bring to a boil, then lower the heat and let it simmer for about 30 minutes, until the lentils are tender.

- Season with salt and pepper, and garnish with fresh parsley before serving.

Mushroom, Garlic, and Parmesan Spaghetti

Ingredients:

- 8 oz spaghetti

- 1 lb fresh mushrooms (like cremini or white)

- 3 cloves garlic, minced

- 1/4 cup grated Parmesan cheese

- Olive oil

- Salt and pepper to taste

- Fresh basil or parsley, for garnish

Procedure:

- Cook the spaghetti according to package instructions. Drain and set aside.

- In the meantime, clean the mushrooms and slice them thinly.

- Heat some olive oil in a pan, add the mushrooms and garlic, and sauté until the mushrooms have released their liquid and are well-cooked.

- Toss the cooked spaghetti with the mushroom mixture. Add the Parmesan cheese and stir well to combine.

- Season with salt and pepper, and garnish with fresh herbs before serving.

Bonus Chapter: The Ancient Use of Medicinal Mushrooms

Mushrooms, found in every corner of the globe, have been both a source of wonder and a wellspring of healing in diverse cultures since time immemorial.

Traditional Chinese Medicine and Medicinal Mushrooms

When we journey to the core of Traditional Chinese Medicine (TCM), it's evident that healing fungi hold a central role. TCM, a health and wellness approach refined across millennia, is inherently linked with the natural environment. Within this complex mosaic, therapeutic mushrooms stand out as vital elements, their benefits deeply rooted in age-old practice and contemporary comprehension.

The conversation around therapeutic mushrooms in TCM wouldn't be complete without acknowledging the esteemed Reishi mushroom, or Lingzhi as it's known in China. Standing as a symbol of long life and wellness, the Reishi has been a part of TCM for over two millennia. Its applications are broad, including fortifying the immune system, aiding cardiovascular health, enhancing mental clarity, and reducing stress. Known as the "Mushroom of Immortality," Reishi embodies the TCM objective of fostering balance between the body, mind, and soul.

Shiitake mushroom is another key component, valued not only for its gastronomic qualities but also for its healing properties. Shiitake has been used in TCM to foster digestion, improve circulation, and boost energy or "Qi". Its bioactive substances, including lentinan, have been extensively researched for their immune-enhancing and anti-cancer properties.

The Cordyceps mushroom, on the other hand, holds a unique position in TCM's history. Referred to as the "winter worm, summer grass" due to its extraordinary lifecycle, Cordyceps is recognized for its ability to increase endurance and combat fatigue. Traditionally, it's been used to bolster kidney and lung health and, more recently, has piqued the interest of athletes and researchers for its potential performance-enhancing properties.

However, the bond between TCM and healing mushrooms transcends utility. In TCM, health isn't merely the absence of disease – it's a state of total equilibrium, a dance between the natural forces of Yin and Yang. Therapeutic mushrooms, with their diverse range of bioactive compounds and health benefits, embody this principle. They are viewed not just as healing agents, but as elements that nourish, harmonize, and align the body with nature's rhythm.

As we persist in investigating the juncture of time-honored wisdom and contemporary science, the use of therapeutic mushrooms in Traditional Chinese Medicine offers a persuasive tribute to nature's enduring role in fostering health and wellness. In a world progressively seeking equilibrium, the teachings from this ancient alliance between therapeutic mushrooms and TCM remain profoundly pertinent.

Ancient European Usage

Exploring the origins of therapeutic mushrooms in European healing traditions propels us on an intriguing voyage into the heart of ancient societies. In these cultures, health and wellness secrets were closely linked to nature. Mushrooms were viewed not just as sustenance, but as crucial partners in their pursuit of comprehensive health.

A fascinating instance of mushroom utilization in ancient Europe is evident in the narrative of Ötzi the Iceman. Found in the Italian Alps, this 5,300-year-old mummy was discovered with two kinds of mushrooms: Birch Polypore and Tinder fungus. Scientists speculate that the Birch Polypore, known for its antiseptic and anti-inflammatory traits, was probably used for medicinal reasons, displaying an early grasp of mushroom curative abilities.

In ancient Greek society, mushrooms held a significant role. Hippocrates, the esteemed physician often considered the progenitor of Western medicine, recognized the Amadou mushroom for its antiseptic and cauterizing properties. In a civilization that established the groundwork for medical rationale and practice, mushrooms were acknowledged as powerful aids in health and disease management.

Progressing to the Middle Ages, medicinal mushrooms continued to be used across European societies. For example, the Agarikon mushroom, celebrated for its potent antibacterial properties, was utilized as 'elixirium ad longam vitam', or the elixir of long life, and was considered a remedy for various ailments, including respiratory illnesses.

European folk medicine traditions also possess a wealth of knowledge about medicinal mushrooms. For instance, Chaga, a fungus indigenous to chilly northern forests, has been brewed into teas by Eastern Europeans for centuries due to its immune-enhancing and overall health-boosting properties.

These glimpses of ancient usage highlight the essential role medicinal mushrooms played in European healing traditions. While the comprehension and use of these mushrooms might have transformed, the fundamental belief remains intact: nature, in its extensive wisdom, presents potent solutions for sustaining health and vigor.

Presently, as scientific exploration illuminates these longstanding practices, we are reminded of the profound wisdom inherent in these traditions. The journey of medicinal mushrooms in Europe attests to human resilience, an enduring fascination with the natural world, and a continuous pursuit of health and wellness. It's a narrative that keeps unfolding, presenting promising prospects for the future of health and medicine.

Medicinal Mushrooms and Native American Healing Practices

Deciphering the connection between therapeutic mushrooms and Native American medicinal traditions is like stepping into a vibrant archive of natural knowledge. Native American tribes have, for innumerable generations, leveraged the healing potency of their environment, seeing health and wellness as a conversation between humans and the world of nature. In this all-embracing perspective, mushrooms emerged as powerful collaborators, with their advantages deeply respected and shared across generations.

The Puffball mushroom stands as one of the most symbolic mushrooms utilized by Native American tribes. Certain tribes harnessed these mushrooms for their properties that promote wound-healing and act as antiseptics. Crushed puffballs were applied directly onto injuries to fend off infection and speed up recovery, illustrating an innate recognition of the antiseptic attributes that we associate with these fungi today.

The Turkey Tail mushroom, recognized for its vivid, fan-shaped appearance akin to a wild turkey's feathers, was also greatly esteemed. Native American tribes immersed these mushrooms in hot water to prepare powerful teas and broths. These concoctions were believed to fortify the immune system and enhance overall vigor, a usage echoed in contemporary research that underscores the mushroom's abundant content of immune-strengthening polysaccharides.

Native Americans also integrated the Reishi mushroom into their healing rituals. This mushroom was consumed as a tonic to foster general health, resilience, and longevity. Its usage was deeply connected to the spiritual and ceremonial life of the tribes, encapsulating the deeply entrenched belief that genuine health includes the physical, emotional, and spiritual aspects of existence.

What distinguishes the Native American utilization of mushrooms is their profound respect for nature. Mushrooms were not merely 'resources' to be exploited, but living entities to be engaged with in a relationship of mutual exchange. This healing approach highlights the importance of balance and harmony with nature, a timeless lesson that remains critically relevant in our present health paradigm.

As we probe further into the intricate world of medicinal mushrooms, the wisdom embedded in Native American healing practices continues to reverberate. Their reciprocal relationship with nature, epitomized in their use of medicinal mushrooms, serves as a compelling reminder of our innate connection to the natural world, and the potential it holds for healing, completeness, and sustainable health.

Modern rediscovery of ancient practices

Nowadays, the curative properties ascribed to therapeutic mushrooms by ancient societies are receiving confirmation through thorough scientific exploration. For instance, the Reishi mushroom, highly valued in Traditional Chinese Medicine, has been found to possess bioactive compounds with anti-inflammatory, immune-regulating, and even anti-cancer effects. In a similar vein, the Turkey Tail mushroom, a common fixture in Native American healing traditions, is presently being investigated for its abundant polysaccharide content, renowned for its immune-enhancing capabilities.

The long-standing use of Chaga in Eastern European traditional medicine serves as another notable illustration. Contemporary research on this medicinal mushroom has identified it as a strong source of antioxidants and anti-inflammatory compounds, corroborating its historic usage for fostering overall wellness and longevity.

This confluence of ancient wisdom and new scientific insight is not simply a validation of old practices but a significant reminder of the applicability of traditional knowledge. It encourages us to re-examine these age-old insights with an attitude of respect and inquisitiveness, acknowledging that they contain practical wisdom that can shape modern health and wellness strategies.

In addition, the current study of medicinal mushrooms offers us something that ancient healers did not have - the technology to deeply examine the molecular structures of these fungi, isolating and comprehending the specific compounds that bestow their health benefits. This, in return, allows for accurate, targeted use in disease treatment and prevention, thereby unveiling a whole new realm of therapeutic potential.

As we persist in investigating the medicinal attributes of mushrooms, we're in many respects simply catching up to what our forebears instinctively grasped. This ongoing journey is a splendid fusion of tradition and innovation, history and science. In this symbiotic dance, we are not only carving out new boundaries in health and medicine but also honouring the enduring wisdom of the past, laying the foundation for a healthier, more balanced future.

Conclusions

As we draw our quest to a close, it is our hope that you have nurtured a fresh reverence and comprehension of mushrooms. Together, we have traversed from the inception of fungi and their role in human chronicles, debunked widespread misunderstandings, and scrutinized the assorted classifications of therapeutic mushrooms. We delved into the prospective advantages of these marvelous organisms in enhancing immunity, mental well-being, anti-aging, gut health, heart health, and their position in cancer deterrence and management.

In the hands-on sections, we have endowed you with the know-how to prepare mushrooms to yield their utmost benefits, comprehend the disparities between supplements and whole mushrooms, and be conscious of potential adverse effects and interactions. Armed with the uncomplicated, nutritious recipes provided, our aspiration is that integrating medicinal mushrooms into your everyday routine will be a health-enhancing decision as much as a flavorful one.

Genuine health and wellbeing stem from a balanced lifestyle encompassing a diverse and nutritious diet, consistent physical activity, ample rest, stress regulation, and a constructive perspective on life. The utilization of medicinal mushrooms should be regarded as a component of a comprehensive strategy for sustaining and enhancing health.

It is our hope that this volume has illuminated your understanding and fortified you with the knowledge to enhance your health in organic and sustainable methods. May your voyage into the captivating universe of medicinal mushrooms perpetually bloom, gifting you health, vitality, and wellness!

www.ingramcontent.com/pod-product-compliance
Lightning Source LLC
Chambersburg PA
CBHW031310250726
48656CB00005B/1726